Praise for Tai Chi Dynamics . . .

Robert Chuckrow has used the insights and experiences gathered from his many years of careful study and teaching of Tai Chi Chuan, physics, and Kinetic Awareness to write a thoughtful, perceptive, open-minded, and at its core, pragmatic approach to the art of Tai Chi Chuan. "I have experienced for *myself* the truth of what I have written," he states in *Tai Chi Dynamics—Principles of Natural Movement, Health, and Self-Development.*

I have often said that I have never been against Tai Chi's "supernatural" elements but prefer to say that I am happy and satisfied with its practical aspects. Robert's book provides Tai Chi practitioners, as well as anyone interested in the dynamics of movement, with many fascinating avenues of practical exploration as a way to discover for themselves the truth Robert writes about.

—*Grandmaster William C.C. Chen,* author
of Body Mechanics of Tai Chi Chuan

It is with great pleasure that I recommend this notable work by my colleague, friend and former classmate, Robert Chuckrow, Ph.D.

Dr. Chuckrow, with his profound knowledge of physics, body mechanics, and Tai Chi Chuan, is in the unusual position of being able to bring his unique perspective to the study of this Chinese exercise and martial art. He analyzes the physical dynamics of the Tai Chi movements in great detail. These insights are particularly relevant to the Western analytical mind.

This book is an important contribution to the body of Tai Chi literature.

—*Lawrence Galante, Ph.D. D.Hom., Director of The Center for
Holistic Arts NYC, author of* Tai Chi: The Supreme Ultimate

In *Tai Chi Dynamics*, Robert Chuckrow adeptly combines his understanding of physics with the principles of Tai Chi. Using simple tools of physics such as inertia, the "pendulum" effect, and conservation of energy to explain Tai Chi movements makes the healing and martial value of Tai Chi more understandable to the modern mind, as it uplifts the science of physics to very practical use.

—*Nancy Rosanoff, auth*

D1403898

Knowing When It's Right

TAI CHI DYNAMICS

Robert Chuckrow, Ph.D.

TAI CHI
DYNAMICS

PRINCIPLES OF NATURAL MOVEMENT, HEALTH, & SELF-DEVELOPMENT

YMAA Publication Center
Boston, Mass. USA

YMAA Publication Center, Inc.
Main Office
23 North Main Street
Wolfeboro, NH 03894
1-800-669-8892 • www.ymaa.com • ymaa@aol.com

© 2008 by Robert Chuckrow

All rights reserved, including the right of reproduction in whole or in part in any form.

Editor: Leslie Takao
Cover Design: Richard Rossiter
Photos by: Ruth Baily, Marian LeConte, Jack Loghry, Nancy Rosanoff, and Kenneth Van Sickle
Illustrations by: Robert Chuckrow and Jizhen Sun Bredeche

ISBN-13: 978-1-59439-116-3
ISBN-10: 1-59439-116-5

10 9 8 7 6 5 4 3 2 1

Publisher's Cataloging in Publication

Chuckrow, Robert.

    Tai chi dynamics : principles of natural
    movement, health, & self-development / Robert
    Chuckrow. -- 1st ed. -- Boston, Mass. : YMAA
    Publication Center, c2008.
        p. ; cm.
        ISBN: 978-1-59439-116-3
        Includes bibliographical references and index.

        1. Tai chi. 2. Health. 3. Mind and body. 4. Self. I. Title.

GV504 .C5363 2008   2008929167
613.7/148--dc22   0806

Warning: Readers are encouraged to be aware of all appropriate local and national laws relating to self-defense, reasonable force, and the use of weaponry, and act in accordance with all applicable laws at all times. Neither the authors nor the publisher assume any responsibility for the use or misuse of information contained in this book.

Nothing in this document constitutes a legal opinion nor should any of its contents be treated as such. While the authors believe that everything herein is accurate, any questions regarding specific self-defense situations, legal liability, and/or interpretation of federal, state, or local laws should always be addressed by an attorney at law.

When it comes to martial arts, self defense, and related topics, no text, no matter how well written, can substitute for professional, hands-on instruction. These materials should be used *for academic study only*.

Printed in Canada.

Dedication

To Elaine Summers, whose genius, generosity in sharing her knowledge, and saint-like patience have given me, among many other things, an understanding of bodily alignment, breathing, stretching, and the distinction between muscular contraction and muscular extension.

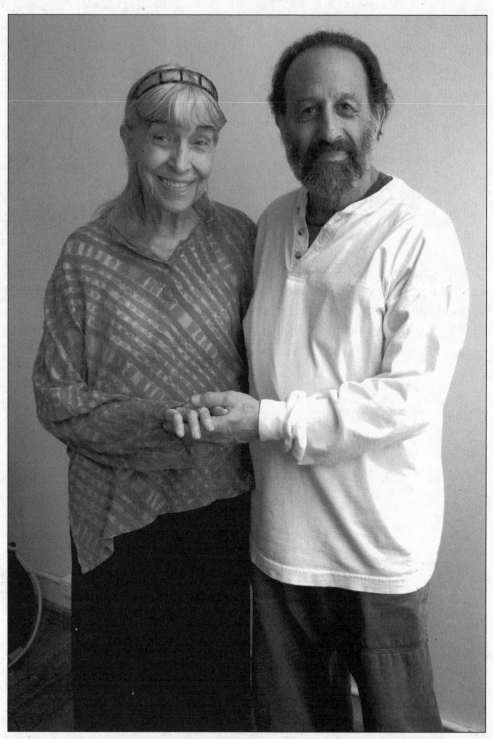

Elaine Summers and the Author. Photograph by Kenneth Van Sickle.

Contents

Administrative Details (Contacting Students who Miss Two or More Classes, Giving Certificates) • Teaching Taiji Push-Hands • Negotiating a Salary when Teaching for Others • Making Changes in the Taiji Form • Monetary Considerations (Vocation or Avocation, How Much to Charge? Charge by the Month or the Series? Payment Policies, Giving Scholarships to Needy Students) • Protecting Yourself (Insurance, Keeping Records, Having Students Sign a Waiver and Release)

Foreword

When two seemingly disparate bodies of knowledge exchange ideas, they both benefit and augment each other. This book exemplifies such an interdisciplinary exchange. Dr. Chuckrow, one of the most inquiring, probing people I know, utilizes his unique gifts of keen perception, love of teaching, and power to connect disciplines. He has studied physics, music, nutrition, Taiji, Qigong, Kinetic Awareness, spiritual teachings, and healing. As a Taiji master and a certified master teacher of Kinetic Awareness, Chuckrow enjoys working to achieve experiential insights. He loves finding the kinetic essentials of a complex Taiji movement and understanding its components. As a physicist, Chuckrow loves the connections that physics brings to understanding the interrelationship between disciplines. One of Chuckrow's great charms is his ability to engage in an intense exploration both verbally and kinetically. He has a searching, perceptive, discovering mind and will wrestle with an idea or insight and strive to connect and understand an idea or experience until it is crystal clear. In this book, which is especially written for intermediate and advanced practitioners, he has used his varied knowledge, organizational skills, and communicative power to translate the language of the body through verbal descriptions and visual images.

Taiji and Kinetic Awareness (KA) are arts that might seem outwardly quite different, but they have a lot in common. Taiji movement is done while upright with only one's feet on the floor, whereas much of KA training involves doing extremely slow and subtle movement, often while lying on balls on the floor. Taiji has its roots in Daoism, applied to movement and self-defense, and KA is a study of the movement of the human body through an understanding of all of its systems. Both arts develop balance, coordination, independence of movement, optimal alignment, reduced susceptibility to injury, and cultivation and utilization of qi. Also, both are systems of health and healing and help with recovery from trauma and ill health.

Elaine Summers, choreographer, filmmaker, inter-media-artist, film-dance & intermedia pioneer. Original member of the Judson Dance Theater.

MA New York University

MIT Fellow (Center for Advanced Visual Studies)

Fulbright Scholar

Originator of Kinetic Awareness

Founder of Experimental Intermedia Foundation

Artistic Director of Elaine Summers Dance & Film Company

Director of the Kinetic Awareness Center

New York, NY

March 19, 2008

Acknowledgments

I am indebted to Elaine Summers, from whom I learned the concept of muscular extension, which is a major theme of this book. I trust that Alice Holtman, a spiritual guide who taught me meditation and healing, would have been pleased with my treatment of that subject matter. Of course, what I have learned from my teachers, Zheng Manqing (Cheng Man-ch'ing), William C.C. Chen, Harvey I. Sober, Kevin Harrington, Michael DeMaio, and Sam Chin Fan-siong, pervades this book. The critical reading of the preliminary manuscript and insightful suggestions of the following people were enormously valuable: Tony Barron, Philip Carter, Sam Chin Fan-siong, Arnold Cohen, Michael Ehrenreich, Michael Fila, Jeffrey M. Fischer, Lawrence Galante, Linda Herko, Marian LeConte, Jack Loghry, Alexis Mohr, Frank Parra, Nancy Rosanoff, Anthony Sciarpelletti, Kenneth Van Sickle, Barbara Smith, Linda Snyder, Harvey I. Sober, and Elaine Summers. I am especially grateful to Jizhen Sun Bredeche for drawing the Chinese characters that appear in this book, to Ken Lara for being my partner for the photographs of the self-defense applications, and to Berty Barranco-Feero, Linda Herko, Marian LeConte, Nancy Rosanoff, Anthony Sciarpelletti, Barbara Smith, and Elly Van Horne for posing for some of the photographs. Finally, I am grateful to Jack Loghry, Nancy Rosanoff, Marian LeConte, and Ruth Baily for taking many of the photographs. I am especially grateful to Kenneth Van Sickle for taking the photograph of Elaine Summers and me.

Author's Background

The Author has been a T'ai-Chi Ch'uan practitioner since 1970 and has studied T'ai Chi under the late Cheng Man-ch'ing, William C. C. Chen, and Harvey I. Sober. He has studied I Liq Ch'uan with Sam Chin Fan-siong, Ninjutsu with Kevin Harrington, Kinetic Awareness with Elaine Summers, and Healing and Re-evaluation with Alice Holtman. He has taught Taiji extensively and has written four other books: *The Tai Chi Book*, *Historical Tuning of Keyboard Instruments*, *The Intelligent Dieter's Guide*, and *Tai Chi Walking*. *The Tai Chi Book* was a finalist in the 1999 Independent Publisher Book Awards as "among the three best books in the health/medicine category."

Chuckrow is certified as a master teacher of Kinetic Awareness, has a Ph.D. in experimental physics from New York University, and has taught Physics at New York University, The Cooper Union, and The Fieldston School in Riverdale, New York.

Author's Note

Every effort has been made to be accurate and helpful. I have experienced for *myself* the truth of what I have written here. However, there may be typographical errors or mistakes in content, or some of the content may not be applicable to everyone. It is my wish that the reader exercise skepticism and caution in applying the information and ideas herein. The purpose of any controversial parts of this book is to stimulate the reader's thinking rather than to serve as an ultimate source of information.

This book is sold with the understanding that neither the author nor publisher is engaged in rendering medical, legal, or other advice; such advice should come from licensed professionals in those respective fields. If medical advice or assistance is required, the services of a competent healthcare professional should be sought. Corresponding statements apply to obtaining advice in other areas. Therefore, neither the author nor publisher shall be held liable or responsible for any harm to anyone from the direct or indirect application of the knowledge, opinions, or ideas expressed herein.

Introduction

Those who study Taiji know that its important concepts are frequently elusive, and, for many practitioners, much of the modern Taiji literature of substantive content is difficult to understand. The pithy written transmissions of the old masters, called *Taijiquan Classics*, tend to be meaningful only *after* one understands their underlying concepts. These transmissions seem to have been intended more for confirming understanding than for imparting it. Originally formulated in Old Chinese, the Taijiquan Classics are very compact and poetic and can be quite mysterious when translated into Modern Chinese and then into English. Old Chinese writing conduced more to self-development than to precision of expression but also served to preserve knowledge for insiders and to keep it inaccessible to outsiders. Consider the following excerpt from the Taijiquan Classics:

> *Every sentence in this thesis is important.*
> *Not a single word has been added carelessly or for decoration.*
> *[Those] without a high degree of wisdom won't be able to understand.*
>
> —Wang, Zong-yue[1]

In China a century or more ago, oral teachings and elucidations of the concepts were essentially reserved for family members. Now, much of the essence of Taiji has been lost or scattered, and serious students often need to study with a succession of teachers, undergo much frustration, and frequently struggle to gain an understanding of the Taiji principles let alone an ability to manifest them.

---

1. Yang, Jwing-Ming, *Tai Chi Secrets of the Ancient Masters*, YMAA Publication Center, Boston, MA, 1999, p. 23.

Of course, much of Taiji needs to be experienced and practiced perseveringly in order to be understood, and words often limit this understanding (a basic Daoist concept).[2] Whereas articulating concepts in a precise, scientific manner cannot provide a complete understanding, doing so can be of much value. It is my hope that my attempts to explain some of the Taiji mysteries by utilizing scientific knowledge, conjecture,[3] distinctions, phraseology, presentation, and approach will help practitioners of this art develop more quickly.

One of the main thrusts of this book is to clarify what is meant by the important concept of *correct strength* (as opposed to *awkward strength*). The concept of correct strength is widely misunderstood but crucial to a number of dimensions of Taiji practice and applications including health, breathing, correct Taiji movement, push-hands, and self-defense. For a long time, I was unable to discern the difference between "correct" and "awkward" strength. My progress was accelerated, however, once I began to apply concepts of physics and anatomy. In an attempt to share my understanding of correct strength, I have presented here an analysis of the anatomical and physiological aspects of muscular action, without which we cannot do *any* voluntary movement including breathing. I have then applied these principles to the two main breathing modalities encountered in Taiji movement, namely, natural breathing and reverse breathing. Finally, I have extended these principles to stepping, shifting weight, turning, and using strength in push-hands and self-defense. In later chapters, I have treated various other subjects including healing, spirituality, and teaching Taiji.

I learned the concepts herein mainly from my teachers Zheng Manqing, Elaine Summers, Alice Holtman, William C.C. Chen, Harvey Sober, Sam Chin Fan-siong, Kevin Harrington, and Michael DeMaio. Over the years, my own practice and reflection, plus the thought-provoking questions that my students have asked me, have helped me to refine what these masters have taught me. In this book, I have simply applied my teaching skills and physics background in attempting to explain and present, in an organized, logical, and scientific manner, the concepts that were taught me.

2. See for example, Lao Tzu: "My words are easy to understand," *Lectures on the Tao Teh Ching by Man-jan Cheng*, Translated by Tam C. Gibbs, North Atlantic Books, 1981.

3. In science, *conjecture* means making an educated guess. Many venerable scientific priciples have originated with conjecture.

Throughout, I have striven not to repeat material covered in my first book, *The Tai Chi Book*, but to use entirely new material and/or presentation. In some cases I have revisited prior material with a new perspective.

Pinyin has been used throughout except for names of historical and other masters, for which use of Wade-Giles is more prevalent. The following table lists some correspondences between the two forms of spelling: [4]

Pinyin	Wade-Giles
Taijiquan	T'ai-Chi Ch'uan
Qi	Ch'i
Qi Gong	Ch'i Kung
Peng	P'eng
Kua	K'ua
Pipa	P'ip'a

---

4. For a useful list of Pinyin/Wade-Giles conversions, see http://library.ust.hk/guides/opac/conversion-tables.html.

1

Muscular Action in Taiji Movement

Two Kinds of Strength

Strength is essential in all martial arts. Without the implied or actual use of physical strength, there is no way that one can defend against a physical attack by a skilled opponent. In fact, without muscular action, no directed movement is possible, not even breathing or circulation of blood. In Taiji, the cultivation and expression of strength are different from that in hard styles such as Karate and Shaolin. Also, Taiji strength is different from the customary strength used in daily life.

My first teacher, Zheng Manqing (Cheng Man-ch'ing),[5] talked about developing "tenacious strength," or "tenacity." According to Zheng, "Tenacity is the resistance or tonicity of living muscles. The muscles being relaxed, tenacity cannot involve the bones. Force, on the other hand, is derived from muscles, binding the bones together into a wooden (rigid) system."[6] Zheng is not alone in making such a distinction; the Taijiquan Classics[7] and other writings frequently mention two corresponding terms, *li* and *jin*. *Li* is translated as *external strength* or *awkward force*, and *jin* is translated as *internal strength* or *correct force*. The character for *li* simply

---

5. See http://www.ibiblio.org/chinesehistory/contents/c06sa01.html for a discussion of the various "Romanizations" of Chinese words (using the English alphabet to write Chinese words).
6. See Cheng Man-ch'ing, *T'ai Chi Ch'uan: A Simplified Method of Calisthenics for Health & Self Defense*, North Atlantic Books, Berkeley, CA, 1981, pp. 16–17.
7. See for example, *The Essence of T'ai-Chi Ch'uan, The Literary Tradition*, Edited by Benjamin Pang-jeng Lo, North Atlantic Books, Berkeley, CA, 1985, pp. 10, 33, 50, 82, 85, 87, 97, and 98.

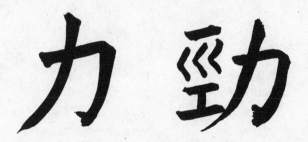

Fig. 1-1. *Left: the character for Li. Right: the character for jin.*

means strength, whereas the character for *jin* means strength that has been refined through experience (jin = li + experience) (see Fig. 1-1). Thus, jin must be cultivated through practice over an extended period of time. Unfortunately, too many Taiji practitioners—even experienced ones—have difficulty in understanding (let alone manifesting) jin, and they incorrectly use li in doing Taiji form and push-hands.[8] Some practitioners use brute strength in doing push-hands, and others are afraid to use force entirely. Both of these extremes prevent practitioners from ever developing jin. In push-hands practice, those who never use strength lose the opportunity to develop jin, and those who use brute strength usually "win" over more-skilled partners, giving them a false impression of success.

The rest of this chapter attempts to analyze muscular action in a way that should reduce the time for practitioners to understand the distinction between jin and li, refine li into jin, and manifest jin everywhere in the body and at any time. The idea will be developed that in Taiji, correct strength originates primarily from muscular extension, in which muscles lengthen (rather than originating from contractive muscular action in which muscles shorten). That is, *jin* will be interpreted as arising from muscular extension, which is unified, is capable of being quickly modified, results in a high level of rootedness,[9] and enhances the flow of qi (ch'i).[10] By contrast, *li* will be interpreted as strength arising primarily

8. Push-hands is a two-person exercise for learning to sense a partner's imbalance and to respond with a carefully timed and placed push that, ideally, will cause one's partner to become airborne. Proper practice of push-hands cultivates balance, root, sensitivity, ego-reduction, and understanding of yin and yang. For a survey of the principles involved, see Robert Chuckrow, *The Tai Chi Book*, YMAA Publication Center, Boston, MA, 1998, Ch. 11.

9. *Rooted* means being connected to the ground like a tree with deep roots and remaining stable despite any manner of force that an opponent tries to exert.

10. For a discussion of qi, see Robert Chuckrow, *The Tai Chi Book*, YMAA Publication Center, Boston, MA, 1998, Ch. 2.

from muscular contraction, which is localized, is difficult to modify with changing conditions, results in balance (root) being relatively easy for an opponent to break, and tends to constrict the flow of qi. Moreover, it will be explained later in this chapter that correct strength is in accord with the balance of yin and yang, whereas incorrect strength is not.

It is not that one form of strength is right in all situations, and the other is wrong. Instead, it is important to recognize the distinction between the two types and be able to use the appropriate combination in a given situation.

FORCE

In physics, *force* is a quantity[11] that distorts the shape of an object or changes its speed or direction of motion. More simply, force can be thought of as a push or pull. Force is measured by the amount of distortion it produces in a standard object such as a spring. Alternatively, force can be measured by noting the resulting acceleration of a standard mass on which the force is exerted; the larger the force, the greater the acceleration. Various units are used in measuring force: The pound is used in England and U.S.A. The kilogram (which really is a measure of mass, not force, but is proportional to the gravitational force on that mass) is used in most other industrialized countries. The catty is traditionally used in China and other Asian countries (1 catty = 1.333 pounds).

The forces that we experience in daily life are either gravitational or electrical. The *weight* of an object is the term used for the familiar gravitational force of attraction by the earth on that object. All other forces that we experience are actually electrical (nuclear forces, which are a third type, are not experienced directly). For example, when you press on a table, the force between the table and your hand is actually the mutual electric repulsion of the outer electrons in the atoms of your hand and those of the surface of the table in "contact" with your hand. *Contact* is in quotes because, microscopically, the atomic particles of the table and hand never actually touch each other but exert repulsive electric forces through small distances. Similarly, electrical forces can cause objects to resist deformation or adhere to other objects.

---

11. In physics, a quantity is anything that can be expressed numerically.

Newton's First Law

It is important to understand Newton's first law, which deals with the behavior of objects in the absence of force:

In the absence of any external force, a stationary object will remain stationary, and a moving object will continue to move at constant speed in a straight line.

Consequently, movement against gravity and changing our motion or that of external objects is impossible without force. The bones in our bodies are moved against gravity only by the forces exerted on them by muscles. Without muscles and the forces they exert, a human body would be unable to move, breathe, or affect its environment physically.

As one trained in physics, I do not disparage the use of force in Taiji but strive to be precise when I discuss it. Understanding how force originates and is applied is of much value. In order to understand correct strength, it is productive to turn to physics, anatomy, and physiology for an understanding of muscular action and a clarification of the distinction between its two kinds, li and jin.

MUSCULAR ACTION: CONTRACTION AND EXTENSION

Whereas the assertions made in this section about muscular extension have not been proven scientifically, my own experience has borne out their validity. I would prefer that the reader neither immediately accept or reject these assertions but keep an open mind. Doing so should open new ways of experiencing Taiji movement and movement in general.

It is generally accepted that muscles are capable of contracting (*muscular contraction*), but few people realize that muscles are also capable of extending (*muscular extension*). I learned about muscular extension from one of my movement teachers, Elaine Summers.[12] This concept has accelerated my progress in Taiji over the past three decades by providing a deeper understanding of Taiji movement, breathing, and use of strength. Here are the two ways that muscles can act:

In the first, familiar mode of muscular action, muscle fibers contract along their length, thereby shortening, making the muscle bulge (see Fig. 1-2).

---

12. Summers uses *extension tension* to refer to what we here call *muscular extension*. The word *tension* in physics refers to the stress resulting from outwardly directed forces applied at opposite ends of the object. An example is a piano string held under tension by pins on each end of the string. To avoid possible confusion, the word *tension* in this discussion has here been avoided when discussing extension.

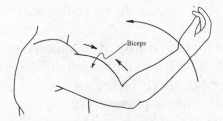 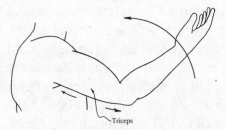

Fig. 1-2. *Muscular contraction of biceps, causing forearm to rotate upward about the elbow. The biceps becomes shorter in length, tightens, and bulges. The arrows above the biceps represent the directions of forces exerted by and movements of the ends of that muscle.*

Fig. 1-3. *The hand extends by means of muscular extension of triceps, causing forearm to rotate upward about the elbow. The biceps becomes shorter in length but stays relaxed. The arrows below the triceps represent the directions of forces exerted by and movements of the ends of that muscle.*

People such as weight-lifters, who cultivate strength primarily through muscular contraction, tend to attain a heavy muscle structure with consequent limited flexibility.

In the second mode of muscular action (about which few people are aware), muscles extend (Fig. 1-3). People who are accustomed to using muscular extension tend to have long, slender muscles.

Summers conjectures that a muscle extends by constricting circumferentially, thereby squeezing the muscle fibers they surround, causing them to elongate (see Fig. 1-4).

Muscular contraction is very strong, and most people use it automatically. However, it can only be sustained for a short period of time because blood supply is constricted and lactic acid builds up quickly, causing the muscle to become fatigued and even painful. Muscular extension, on the other hand, takes some training to recognize and develop. Once developed, however, muscular extension can also be strong. But unlike muscular contraction, muscular extension can be

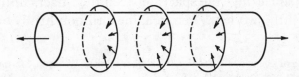

Fig. 1-4. *Possible circular constriction of muscle fibers, causing axial lengthening of the muscle composed of those fibers. The horizontal cylinder represents a bundle of muscle fibers, and the circles represent the direction of constriction of that bundle, elongating it.*

maintained for relatively long periods of time because lactic acid builds up more slowly and is more easily dissipated.

Zheng Manqing was able to stably maintain the "Ward Off" stance with four strong students pushing his extended arm.[13] He could manifest this kind of rooting and expansive strength, called *peng jing*,[14] in the last years of his life. Zheng was slight of build and certainly was not physically strong in the conventional sense (li).[15] There is little doubt that Zheng was using muscular extension to accomplish this feat.

Whereas we are not accustomed to using muscular extension deliberately, we do use it whenever we reach for something, yawn, or stretch naturally (as opposed to the kind of stretching often done in exercise classes). Unnatural stretching involves using one set of muscles and leverage to force the opposing set of muscles to lengthen. Natural stretching occurs when the muscles to be lengthened do so on their own, by muscular extension. Therefore, it should not be difficult to recognize that muscles *are* capable of extending. Once you recognize the feeling accompanying muscular extension, you can capture it and then practice recreating it. The following are exercises for achieving such recognition.

Exercises for Recognizing: Muscular Extension

Exercise 1. Try yawning—recreating the feeling throughout your body of the most intense yawn you ever experienced. Then sustain that open, extended state in the musculature of the trunk of your body and arms, and, at the same time, relax the musculature of the jaw, trachea, and ribs. The state you will be in is that of muscular extension (correct force). Now capture that feeling, and practice recreating it until you can bring it to Taiji or Qigong movements consistently.

Exercise 2. Stand with feet parallel and knees somewhat bent. Let the one arm hang naturally. Extend the other arm in front of your body at a comfortable level. Relax the extended arm and hand as much as possible. Start by gently "squeezing" the space between the fingers until the hand starts to feel slightly swollen. Then imagine a ribbon firmly but gently

---

13. For a photograph of Zheng demonstrating this skill, see Robert W. Smith, *Martial Musings*, Via Media Publishing Company, Erie, PA, 1999, p. 288.

14. For a discussion of *pengjin* (expansive strength resulting from jing), see http://www.taiji-qigong .de/info/articles/jumin_transljin_en.php.

15. For more on Zheng Manqing, see Robert W. Smith, *Martial Musings: A Portrayal of Martial Arts in the 20th Century*, Via Media Publishing Company, Erie, PA, 1999. This book has many anecdotes about Zheng. Smith is an accomplished martial artist and was a close student of Zheng.

wrapped around your forearm, starting at the elbow and winding to the wrist (experiment with the direction that it wraps). Create a state inside your arm wherein you are gently squeezing the way the ribbon would. Feel your fingers as you continue to squeeze. Then, use that feeling to extend your hand forward. You should now be experiencing muscular extension. Sustaining this state, wrap an imaginary ribbon around your upper arm. Continue to experiment with gentle extension of the hand.

Next, change the previous action to one of contraction, and note the difference in feeling. Alternate between contraction and extension until you can readily recognize and recreate muscular extension. When you start to tire, slowly lower your arm until it hangs by your side. Compare the feeling in the two arms. Then repeat the entire exercise with the other arm.

A Reconsideration of Zheng's Distinction Between the Two Types of Strength

Let us now reconsider Zheng's statement, mentioned earlier in this chapter: "Tenacity is the resistance or tonicity of living muscles. The muscles being relaxed, tenacity cannot involve the bones. Force, on the other hand, is derived from muscles, binding the bones together into a wooden (rigid) system." When you achieve the ability to move and exert force on another person by means of muscular extension, it will feel as though you have no bones. Moreover, your muscles will feel relaxed because they are not in a state of familiar muscular contraction. When you change to muscular contraction, you will immediately feel the muscles in a state of contraction and the tendons exerting large forces on the bones. You will also feel a "wooden" rigidity that pervades the body beyond that of the limb being used.

UNIFIED STRENGTH AND PASCAL'S PRINCIPLE

"Unified strength" is so called because it involves every part of the body instead of involving a localized expression of strength. When the whole body becomes devoid of contractive muscular action, it behaves somewhat like a confined liquid; after all, our bodies are composed of 90% water. Then, when all muscle groups are activated through muscular extension, a sort of hydraulic pressure builds up in the body, which connects every part to every other part. This pressure is felt especially in the dan tian.[16] According to Pascal's principle, an increase in pressure at any point in a confined liquid results in an equal increase in pressure at every other point. That is, pressurizing one region of the body through muscular extension causes every other region to become likewise pressurized. This pressure permeates every part of the body, and an increase in pressure at any point can be used to move any other part of the body. The result is the ability to express very large force at any point in any direction, and this strength comes from the ground, thereby rooting the whole body. The implication of Pascal's principle is basically equivalent to the saying that when one part moves, every part moves:

> *Remember, when moving, there is no place that doesn't move.*
> —Wu Yu-hsiang[17]

IMPLIED STRENGTH

At each moment, every part of the body must have implied strength in every direction. Implied strength is a state of unified, subtle muscular extension throughout the whole body. In this state, the implied strength can escalate in intensity at will and at a moment's notice. In this state, the awareness encompasses every part of the body involved and the intensity of the muscular extension involved.

By practicing unified strength in Qigong and in the Taiji form, you will attain "correct strength," enhanced flow of qi, beautifully coordinated movement, and a state of heightened sensitivity to and awareness of another's intention.

---

16. The dan tian is a region centered about an inch below the navel, one-third of the way from front to back. The Japanese refer to that region as *hara*. The dan tian is the center of gravity of the body and is the region where qi is said to be stored.

17. *The Essence of T'ai Chi Ch'uan, The Literary Tradition*, Edited by Benjamin Pang-jeng Lo et al., North Atlantic Books, Berkeley, CA, 1985, p. 57.

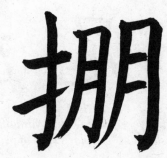

Fig. 1-5. *The character for peng. The radical (on the left) represents hand, and the two characters on the right represent two moons. The presence of two adjacent reflecting objects suggests the idea of mutual repulsion or outward, expansive strength.*

PENG

Peng is the upward and outward movement resulting from unified, muscular extension. The cultivation of peng usually requires years of doing push-hands and practicing the Taiji empty-hand form. Perhaps the following discussion will shorten the time to recognize and manifest peng.

As you start to pronounce the word *peng* (pronounced *pung*), before your lips begin to open, you will feel air pressure building up in your mouth and lungs. This pressure is a result of the expansion of the diaphragm (muscular extension). Whatever the derivation of the character for peng (Fig. 1-5), just saying *peng* suggests the feeling of using muscular extension to create hydraulic pressure to express an outward and upward expansive strength.

The Chinese characters that name the movements in the Taiji form, "Ward off Left," and "Ward off Right" actually include the final character *peng* (see Fig. 1-6).[18] In each of these movements, an arm rises upward and outward from waist level. In both the original Yang form and in Zheng's 37-posture form, these movements occur right after the "Beginning" movement. In the newer, 24-posture Beijing form, the ward-off movements at the beginning are replaced by left and right styles of "Parting the Wild Horse's Mane." These latter movements are very similar to and in the same category as the ward-off movements. Both "Ward off" and "Parting the Wild Horse's Mane" involve an upward and outward sweep of an arm. That these movements incorporating peng appear right after the beginning

---

18. See Cheng Man-ch'ing, *T'ai Chi Ch'uan: A Simplified Method of Calisthenics for Health & Self Defense*, North Atlantic Books, Berkeley, CA, 1981, p. 46.

攬 雀 尾 左 掤

Fig. 1-6. *The characters Lan Que Wei Zuo Peng for "Ward off Left," which include the character peng and can be translated as "circular sweep of peacock's tail left peng."*

movement of the form suggests the importance of cultivating the correct muscular action required to do these movements properly. Actually, all Taiji movements (up, down, right, left, in, and out) require peng in order to be done properly, but the ward-off movements display peng visibly. The following are two exercises for attaining peng.

Exercises for Recognizing Peng

Exercise 1. (See Fig. 1-7.) Player *A* (on the right) stands in the "Ward Off Left" posture, and player *B* (on the left) stands facing *A* in the "Push" posture. The hollow of *B*'s right hand centers on *A*'s left elbow, and that of her left hand centers on *A*'s right wrist joint. Each of *B*'s hands gently touch *A* but exert practically no force. *A* relaxes his shoulder, elbow, wrist, etc., as much as possible. *B*'s job is to detect any contractive tension in *A* and help him relax it. Once *A* is as relaxed as possible, he starts to expand into *B*'s hands almost imperceptibly. When *B* feels *A*'s expansion, she maintains increasing pressure only in the amount that prevents *A* from moving. Gradually, mutual pressure builds up from mutual extension rather than from contraction. As soon as either player notices any contractive force, both players reduce their mutual force until muscular contraction subsides. Next *A* and *B* swap roles.

Exercise 2. This exercise does not require a partner. Stand in the "Ward Off Left" posture, with your forearm against a wall. After concentrating on relaxing without exerting any force on the wall, gradually build up force, being careful not to revert to muscular contraction. This latter exercise does not require a partner but lacks a partner's feedback.

Once the feel of peng is captured, the next step is to incorporate it into meditative one-handed push-hands as follows:

Exercise 3. Let your ankle, knee, and hip joints be very relaxed. As your partner pushes on your wrist, use peng to keep the arm from collapsing even a little bit. However, to the extent that the ankle, knee, and hip joints are very loose, it will take only a small force for your partner to move you back. When you are being pushed, you should be yin, not yang. Therefore, your movement is passive, not active, which means that pulling back, which is yang (active), would violate the principle of yin and yang.

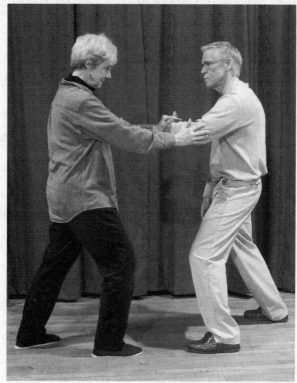

Fig. 1-7. *An exercise for recognizing peng.*

Many push-hands practitioners develop contractive force to a large degree and are able to use it effectively against less-skilled partners. However, the success such practitioners experience is a developmental dead end. On the other hand, your willingness to temporarily "lose" at push-hands and your persistence in developing peng will be well worth the time and effort required.

> *From familiarity with the correct touch, one gradually understands chin [jin] (internal force); from the comprehension of chin, one can reach wisdom.*
>
> —Wang Tsung-yueh[19]

Allowing your partner's force to move you ensures (a) that you are satisfying yin and yang and (b) that you are moving in accordance with your partner's movements and not from your own preconception of how and when to move. Minimizing the force required by your partner to move you also teaches you to release your knee, thigh, and ankle joints. However, after

---

19. *The Essence of T'ai Chi Ch'uan, The Literary Tradition,* Edited by Benjamin Pang-jeng Lo et al., North Atlantic Books, Berkeley, CA, 1985, p. 40.

this manner of movement is perfected, there are two more elements that come into play in push-hands practice. One is having your partner's intention move you, and the other is *leading* your partner into his/her weakness, that is, always seeming to be within easy reach and susceptible to being pushed but always just beyond reach, causing your partner to overextend. Of course, having your partner's intention move you and *leading* your partner into weakness can only be developed after you rid yourself of awkward strength and of impulsive, disconnected, discontinuous responses.

Muscular Action and Yin and Yang

When a limb moves away from the body, its action can be considered to be yang (upward, outward, expansive, active, etc.). To balance yin and yang, the supporting structures of the active limb must, therefore, be yin (supportive, inactive). When a limb moves by contractive muscular action, the reaction to the muscular force that pulls the limb is a lifting pull on the other end of the supporting structure. Thus, moving or exerting force by using muscular contraction, pulls the body out of its root, thus preventing it from being yin (the supporting structures must be active to pull back). That is why, when the object on which force is exerted gives way, the person exerting the force loses his/her root and falls forward.

On the other hand, when a limb moves by muscular extension, the reaction (*see Newton's Third Law in Ch. 4*) to the muscular force that pushes the limb is an inward push on the other end of the supporting structure. Moving or exerting force by using muscular extension pushes the body into its root and makes it more yin (ultimately, the ground provides the support). That is why, when the object on which force is exerted gives way, the person exerting force by using muscular extension does not lose his/her root—in fact the root increases.

Sympathetic Muscular Tension

It is common for the untrained person to exert force inefficiently. Breathing becomes restricted, shoulders rise when a hand is lifted, and tension appears in the upper body when stepping. That is, a muscular action is often accompanied by a sympathetic, inappropriate array of unnecessary tension in the body. As training progresses and jin replaces li, efficiency improves. For example, once you achieve correct jin, you can stand in the "Ward-Off" posture and allow a strong person to push on your outstretched arm and still have your wrist, hand, and fingers be totally soft.

2

Breathing in Taiji

T here is no one way to breathe for Taiji practice (or in daily life for that matter). Moshé Feldenkrais said the following during a weekend workshop I attended in 1973: "The function of breathing is much more complex than what you see. To breathe correctly means at least fifty different types of breathing. If you breathe in love-making like you breathe now, you need another partner. Each act needs a special kind of breathing. Just as I can't teach you what to say, you can't breathe the way someone teaches you." That is, the basic idea of breathing exercises is not to teach you how to breathe but to introduce your body to a variety of ways of breathing. Then, your natural breathing will likely be more appropriate in a given situation.

It is very beneficial for the Taiji practitioner to be proficient in and understand the physiology of both natural and reverse breathing because each method has unique and complimentary benefits. What follows is an attempt to clarify the differences between these two modalities and some of their respective benefits.

Note: Please do not be discouraged should it take a few readings of this chapter to understand it. It took me years of asking my teachers questions, consulting anatomy books, and devoting much thought and practice before I sufficiently understood what I present here. Give it some time, and you will not be sorry.

NATURAL BREATHING

Natural breathing refers to the way we would breathe in the absence of (a) any Yogic or other training of breathing and (b) any encumbrances to

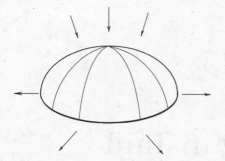

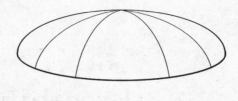

Fig. 2-1. *During an inhalation in natural breathing, the diaphragm expands circumferentially, causing it to flatten. The direction of each arrow represents the direction of motion of the edge or surface from which it points toward or away.*

Fig. 2-2. *After an inhalation in natural breathing, the diaphragm is in the circumferentially expanded and flattened shape shown (here greatly exaggerated).*

breathing such as restrictive clothing, a history of smoking, being overweight, exposure to air pollution, etc.

In natural breathing, both the ribs and diaphragm work together. Recall that the diaphragm is a domed, circular, sheet-like muscle whose circumference lies at the base of the ribs. Please note that the diaphragm attaches at the bottom of the sternum in the front of the body and at the base of the ribs in the back. Thus, the dome faces diagonally upward, toward the back of the body—not vertically upward, as shown for simplicity in the accompanying figures.

Inhalation. During an inhalation, the diaphragm widens circumferentially outward (muscular extension) causing it to flatten downward (see Figs. 2-1 and 2-2). The ribs respond to the widening of the circumference of the diaphragm by expanding outward. Of course, the downward movement of the diaphragm during inhalation also compresses the region below it, causing the lower abdomen to expand. Both the outward bellows-like action of the ribs and the piston-like flattening of the diaphragm cause air to be drawn into the lungs to fill what is now a larger cavity in the rib cage. Note that for an inhalation that is more complete than occurs in natural breathing, the muscles that activate the movement of the ribs must use muscular extension.

Exhalation. During an exhalation, the diaphragm relaxes, causing it to become increasingly domed and smaller in circumference (see Fig. 2-3). The ribs, in turn, relax inward to a neutral position. Both of these actions

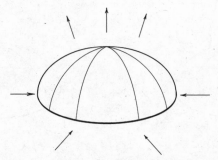

Fig. 2-3. *During an exhalation in natural breathing, the diaphragm relaxes inward circumferentially and upward, assuming its neutral domed shape.*

cause air to be expelled from the lungs. Note that for an exhalation that is more complete than occurs in natural breathing, the muscles that activate the movement of the ribs must use muscular contraction.

Unfortunately, many people have no training and have been exposed to factors that affect breathing negatively. Consequently, they breathe shallowly, barely activating their diaphragms at all. Such shallow breathing deprives the organs, blood vessels, nerves, acupuncture meridians, and muscles in the abdomen of an important periodic massage.

REVERSE BREATHING

Reverse breathing is aptly named because it is essentially the reverse of natural breathing. In reverse breathing, the diaphragm is gently kept expanded circumferentially. This action flattens the diaphragm, increasing its surface area and creating a pressure build-up in the lower abdomen. Moreover, the rib cage is kept slightly expanded, passively, by the action of the diaphragm.

Exhalation. During an exhalation, the diaphragm *stays expanded circumferentially and, by means of muscular extension,* expands upward (becomes more domed) (see Fig. 2-4). In order for the diaphragm to expand upward, it must be supported circumferentially. Thus, the exhalation causes the edges of the diaphragm to exert a downward and outward pressure along the entire circumference (front, sides, and rear) of the diaphragm.

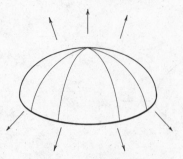

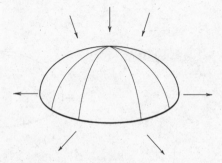

Fig. 2-4. *During an exhalation in reverse breathing, the diaphragm expands downward and outward circumferentially and expands upward, becoming more domed.*

Fig. 2-5. *During an inhalation in reverse breathing, the diaphragm expands circumferentially and relaxes downward, becoming less domed.*

We all are proficient at doing the exhalation part of reverse breathing when exerting a large force on an external object or during a sneeze, cough, or shout. To help recognize what occurs in reverse breathing, try voluntarily coughing while placing the web of each of your hands called *tiger's mouth* (*Hu Kou*) (thumbs in back) around the circumference of your diaphragm. You should be able to feel the reaction force with your hands. Simply stated, the only way to expel air forcibly is by muscular action (in this case expansion). *Exhaling by contracting the ribcage and relaxing the diaphragm will not produce the required power!*

Inhalation. The inhalation involves a release of the upward (but not circumferential) expansion of the diaphragm (see Fig. 2-5), causing it to flatten, thus drawing air into the lungs. In reverse breathing the ribs have only minor movement.

EXERCISES FOR RECOGNIZING DIAPHRAGMATIC EXTENSION

Exercise 1. Stand in a relaxed manner. With your wind pipe gently sealed with the back of your tongue, create air pressure in your lungs using your diaphragm. This action will expand your diaphragm by means of muscular extension. The feeling of diaphragmatic expansion is the same as that in reverse breathing. Next, let the compressed air in your lungs escape. When you release your diaphragm, you will notice that air will automatically enter your lungs.

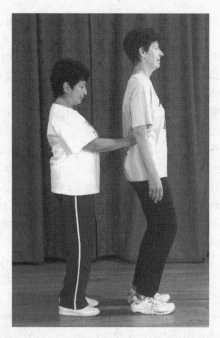

Fig. 2-6. *Here, a student is using her hands to sense the action of another student's diaphragm and offering verbal feedback.*

Exercise 2. *B* stands behind *A* with the webs of her hands, which are palm-down, circling *A*'s diaphragm (see Fig. 2-6). It is *A*'s job to expand her diaphragm circumferentially while *B* offers feedback by the resistance of her touch and her verbal comments. Then *A* and *B* swap roles.

YIN AND YANG OF NATURAL BREATHING CONTRASTED TO THAT OF REVERSE BREATHING

When doing natural breathing, the inhalation is the active part (muscular action) and the exhalation is the passive part (muscular release). Thus, the yang part of natural breathing is the inhalation. On the other hand, when doing reverse breathing, the exhalation is the active part and the inhalation is the passive part. Thus, the yang part of reverse breathing is the exhalation. These differences have important ramifications in Qigong and self-defense. Table 2-1, later in this chapter, summarizes these and other aspects of natural and reverse breathing.

Advantages of Natural Breathing in Taiji and Qigong

When doing Taiji or Qigong solely for health or during the initial stages of learning, the main emphasis should be on relaxing the whole body and on strengthening the legs. Contractive muscular action cuts off qi and makes movement awkward. It also brings the center of gravity higher. Therefore, during each transition of Taiji or Qigong, an exhalation by releasing (natural breathing) allows the deepest state of relaxation of the trunk of the body down into the legs (as in sitting down into a chair after a hard day's work). An inhalation during a completed posture oxygenates the body and stimulates the flow of qi. It is not hard to experience that qi increases during an inhalation and decreases during an exhalation.

An opportunity to verify the oxygenating effect of breathing occurs when you have a cut, bruise, sprain, etc. It has been my experience that the pain of such an injury increases during an exhalation and decreases during an inhalation. These effects of breathing on qi and pain strongly suggest that qi is interconnected with the oxygenation of bodily tissues and possibly also by the muscular extension accompanying an inhalation.

Natural breathing requires nothing special to learn and, therefore, is ideal for beginners struggling to learn such a complex and elusive art as Taiji. This consideration may be the reason that some Taiji teachers who are adept at reverse breathing solely teach natural breathing to beginners.

Advantages of Reverse Breathing in Taijiquan and Qigong

The use of reverse breathing is very important for advanced practitioners and, especially, for those who emphasize the martial (*quan*)[20] aspects of Taiji. The implied or actual exertion of any large force on an external object or on another person must involve connecting the upper and lower parts of the body. If the upper and lower parts of the body are too loosely connected, any attempt to exert force will result in the body flexing, thus reducing the amount of force that can be exerted. The connection between the upper and lower parts of the body is greatly augmented by the diaphragmatic action of a forceful exhalation. Thus, in all martial arts, strikes

---

20. The Chinese word *quan* (Ch'uan) literally means *fist*, so *Taijiquan* (T'ai-Chi Ch'uan) usually refers to the practice of Taiji for martial skill.

and kicks are accompanied by an exhalation using reverse breathing. In fact, in some arts, the exhalations accompanying certain strikes are voiced (*kiai*). Karate practitioners contract their skeletal muscles during a strike or kick; nevertheless, the forcible exhalation cannot occur without muscular extension of the diaphragm.

During Taiji-form practice, even if the forceful exhalation and its application are only implied, the expansive action of the diaphragm in reverse breathing helps to cultivate increasingly stronger correct force. Just as contractive tension in one part of the body tends to produce a sympathetic corresponding tension in other parts, using muscular extension in one part conduces to its sympathetic spread to other parts. At the very least, we are good at using muscular extension for breathing, and doing so prompts it to spread to other parts of the body.

Another aspect of reverse breathing is that its expanded-diaphragm state enhances the flow of qi. Moreover, the flattening of the diaphragm by expanding it circumferentially in reverse breathing both pressurizes the lower abdomen (*dan tian*) and forces more oxygen into the bloodstream than does natural breathing. Further, reverse breathing helps create an internal hydraulic pressure, which makes the body resilient and strong.

Thus, reverse breathing adds important dimensions to Taiji movement in *both* the strength and health realms. Advanced practitioners should practice both types of breathing (not during the same form, of course) to balance their benefits.

Table 2-1. A summary of primary advantages and aspects of natural and reverse breathing.

	Natural Breathing	*Reverse Breathing*
Qi Enhancement	✓	✓
Martial Power		✓
Strength of Legs	✓	
Relaxation	✓	
Inhalation	Yang	Yin
Exhalation	Yin	Yang
Final Postures	Inhalation	Exhalation
Transitions	Exhalation	Inhalation

Coordination of Breathing with Movement in Taiji Practice when Utilizing Natural Breathing

When doing natural breathing, during an upward and outward movement of the arms, it is natural to breathe in, and during a downward and inward movement of the arms, it is natural to breathe out. So, for example, in doing "Ward Off Left," as the weight shifts onto the right foot and the two hands form a ball-holding position, one would breathe out. After stepping with the left foot, as the weight shifts to that foot and the left hand rises to mid-chest level, one would breathe in. Thus, when doing the Taiji movements using natural breathing, the final postures involve an inhalation, and the transitions involve an exhalation.

It should be kept in mind that practicing the Taiji movements using natural breathing is more for cultivating relaxation and strength of legs (rooting) than for developing martial power.

Coordination of Breathing with Movement in Taiji Practice when Utilizing Reverse Breathing

When doing Taiji using reverse breathing, during an upward and outward movement, one breathes out, and during a downward and inward movement, one breathes in ("condensing"). So, for example, in doing "Ward off Left," as the weight shifts onto the right foot and the two hands form a ball-holding shape, one breathes in. After stepping with the left foot, as the weight shifts to that foot and the left hand rises to mid-chest level, one breathes out. Thus, when doing the Taiji movements using reverse breathing, the final postures involve an exhalation, and the transitions involve an inhalation.

It should be kept in mind that practicing the Taiji movements for cultivating martial power, one must use reverse breathing. However, even if you are mainly interested in cultivating relaxation and strength of the legs, it is also good but not necessary to occasionally do the Taiji form using reverse breathing, whose pressurizing effect has an important benefit of augmenting the flow and experiencing of qi.

CONTRASTING DIFFERENT MASTERS'
BREATHING INSTRUCTIONS

Some highly accomplished Taiji masters emphasize not doing any specialized breathing, whereas others consider specialized breathing to be crucial. Zheng told us that in the "Beginning" movement, one breathes in as the hands rise, and in the rest of the movements, "breathing takes care of itself." When teaching beginners, William C.C. Chen emphasizes natural breathing in every movement of the form, and in his books and classes, he specifies exactly when one should breathe in and when one should breathe out.[21] Sam Chin Fan-siong teaches reverse breathing and also specifies exactly when one should breathe in and when one should breathe out. Harvey Sober considers breathing to be of utmost importance. He once said that in every fighting competition he won, it was because his opponent did not breathe correctly. Sober teaches many different types of breathing but, like Zheng, never suggests any hard-and-fast rule about breathing during form practice. After being exposed to all the different ways, the body should find its own way in each situation.

Of course, it is possible that Zheng refrained from teaching us specialized breathing until we were more advanced and died before having a chance to teach it. It is also probable that Chen teaches reverse breathing to his top students after a certain point in their development. His ability to "take punches"[22] must require him to do reverse breathing.

It is almost inconceivable that anyone can become expert in Taiji without any breathing instruction.

FOUR BREATHING EXPERIMENTS

I was taught the following experiments separately (but slightly differently) by Moshé Feldenkrais and Elaine Summers. These experiments are best done while lying quietly on your back on the floor.

---

21. See William C. C. Chen, *Body Mechanics of T'ai Chi Ch'uan*, William C. C. Chen Publisher, New York, NY, 1973, and William C. C. Chen, "William C. C. Chen on Tai Chi Breathing," *T'ai Chi Magazine*, December, 2006, pp. 6–11.
22. William C.C. Chen is renown for his ability to be unharmed by powerful strikes to just about any part of his body.

Experiment 1. Breathe in fully. Exhale keeping the diaphragm expanded—front, sides, and rear. With each successive inhalation, expand the diaphragm even more.

Experiment 2. Breathe in fully. Exhale keeping the ribs expanded. With each successive inhalation, expand the ribs even more.

Experiment 3. Breathe out completely. Inhale keeping the lower abdomen constricted, which prevents the action of the diaphragm. With each successive exhalation, constrict the lower abdomen even more.

Experiment 4. Breathe out completely. Inhale keeping the ribs constricted. With each successive exhalation, constrict the ribs even more.

The discomfort in doing these four exercises stems from disconnecting the usual link between the actions of the ribs and those of the diaphragm. Moreover, these exercises show that link but also that these actions are not *totally* linked. Experiments of this sort break up habitual breathing patterns, exercise the musculature of breathing, oxygenate the body, and stimulate neural pathways and processing. All of these features pave the way to breathing more appropriately when no thought is given to the processes.

A Story

When I was studying with William C. C. Chen in the mid 1970s, I often arrived early to warm up and stretch. One day, I came to a studio that was empty except for an elderly Chinese gentleman standing in the center of the room. I immediately recognized him to be T. T. Liang. I said hello and, after a while, approached him saying, "Can I ask you a question? He answered, "I'm retired" and waved me away. I said, "The question is about qi." He said, "What's qi?" I tried my best to give him an answer even though I realized that he was playing with me. Next he said, "Put your hands on my waist." He powerfully expanded his whole waist area—front, back and sides. Then he said, "learn that," and walked away.

I practiced what he had told me to do every day. When I sewed shoes by hand, for each stitch, I used the expansion of my lower abdomen to push the awl through the leather. After each stitch, I placed the awl in a different location on my abdomen.

It was only years later that I realized that the action he showed me was the expansion of the diaphragm in reverse breathing.

SUSPENDING BREATHING COMPARED TO HOLDING THE BREATH

People tend to hold their breath when confronted with a stressful situation. Of course, holding the breath actually makes it harder to deal with stress because of the lack of exchange of carbon dioxide and oxygen and the unnecessary muscular action, both of which *increase* the need for oxygen.

Suspending breathing is quite different and is a natural phenomenon. At times, the need for oxygen is absent for a while, and one can enjoy relaxing and not having to breathe for a fraction of a minute. This state is one of relaxation and an appropriate response to the lack of a need to breathe. Such a state is probably similar to that of a normal fetus in the womb, where breathing is not continuous but is intermittent, stopping for periods of up to 20 seconds.[23]

HICCUPS

Hiccups result from spasms of the diaphragm. Next time you suffer from hiccups, try the following remedy, which in my experience, always works: All that is needed is to suspend breathing (not holding one's breath but staying relaxed and just not breathing) for about 30 seconds. The short rest given the diaphragm is usually sufficient.

---

23. See *http://www.emedicine.com/ped/byname/apnea-of-prematurity.htm.*

3

Relationships of Conditions, Shape, Timing, Muscular Action, and Yin and Yang in Taiji Movements

RELATIVE MOTION

In order to discuss the movement of a part of the body without ambiguity, it is necessary to specify the frame of reference in which the movement is viewed. For example, saying that the head does not move can have more than one meaning: One meaning is that the head does not move relative to the body, which *may be* moving. Another meaning is that the head is not moving in space, which might occur if the body is turning about an axis with the head fixed in space and always facing the same direction. Being clear about the frame of reference aids our communication with others and adds a dimension of understanding to our own movement. Beyond specifying the frame of reference, it is necessary to state direction (up, down, right, left, forward, back, and clockwise or counterclockwise about a specified axis).

PLANES OF THE BODY

Because the space in which we move is three-dimensional, any movement can be specified by its components of motion in each of three mutually perpendicular planes (median, frontal, or horizontal). The median plane is a vertical plane that separates the body into right-and-left symmetrical halves (*median = middle*). The frontal plane is a vertical plane that divides front and back (or here, any plane parallel to it). The horizontal plane is a level plane (see Fig. 3-1). During movement, the median and frontal planes move with the body. Thus, movement described in the frontal and median planes is relative to the body. Also of value is the sagittal plane, which is any plane parallel to the median plane.

An example of how motion can be described in terms of the three planes, consider the transition from "Push" to "Single Whip" in Zheng Manqing's style. As you sit back from "Push," both hands move forward (relative to the body), each in a sagittal plane. Then, the right hand moves counterclockwise in a horizontal plane during the rest of the transition. After moving sagittally, the left hand first moves counterclockwise in a horizontal plane, then counterclockwise in a frontal plane until it reaches face level. Then, it moves counterclockwise in a horizontal plane and

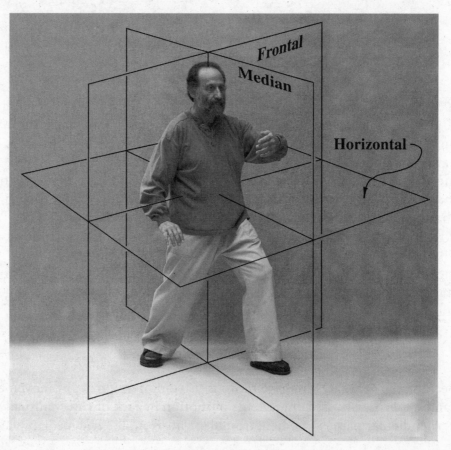

Fig. 3-1. *The frontal, horizontal, and median planes of the body.*

simultaneously rotates clockwise about the axis of the arm until it faces forward. The left wrist ends up in front of left shoulder. Other styles have other ways of doing "Single Whip." For example, Kwong Yung-cheng (Franklin Kwong), a classmate of Zheng Manqing under Yang Cheng-fu, did this transition as follows: As you sit back from "Push," both hands move counterclockwise in a large circle in a frontal plane. When the right hand reaches waist level, it forms the "bird's beak" and moves upward and away from the body to an extended position at shoulder level. The left hand continues its counterclockwise motion in a frontal plane until it is in front of the face. Then it moves counterclockwise in a horizontal plane and simultaneously rotates clockwise about the axis of the arm until it faces forward, wrist in front of left shoulder.

Of course, movement can be simultaneously in more than one plane. In the transition from "Beginning" into "Ward off Left," the left hand first moves in the frontal plane. Then, as that hand sweeps upward and outward, it moves in both the frontal and median planes.

DEGREE OF FREEDOM

The number of degrees of freedom of a part of the body is the number of independent ways that body part can move. For example, the head can tilt side to side (move frontally), tilt forward and backward (move medially), or turn side to side (about a vertical axis). To a small extent, the head can move up and down (vertically). Thus the head can be said to have three degrees of freedom (four if we stretch things). All movement of the head can be described in terms of individual movements corresponding to each of these degrees of freedom. When the motion of two or more parts of the body are described together, the number of degrees of freedom add numerically.

As another example, an arm can swing vertically, horizontally, extend along its length, and rotate about its length. Thus, the arm has four degrees of freedom.

Awareness of the degrees of freedom of a part of the body helps in ensuring the integrity of its movement.

PARALLAX

Parallax is the apparent relative movement of two objects at different distances from an observer, resulting from movement of the observer. Simply stated, when you focus on a distant object and move your head in one direction, the closer object will appear to move in the opposite direction.

Experiment 1. View a distant building through a window. While looking at the building, move your head to the left, and notice that the vertical sash bars and window frame will appear to move to the right (see Fig. 3-2). Similarly, while looking at the building, move your head upward, and notice that the horizontal sash bars and window frame will appear to

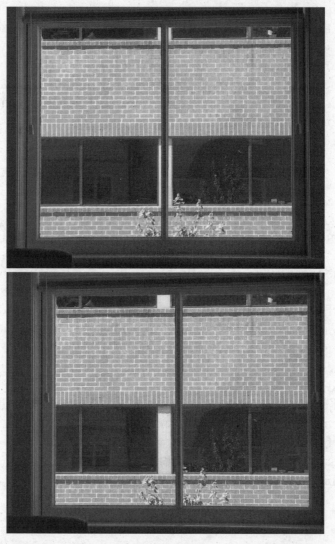

Fig. 3-2. *Two photographs taken of a brick building through a window. The photo on the bottom was taken with the camera moved several inches to the left of its position for the photo on the top but remaining centered on the building window.*

move downward. Similar statements apply to moving your head to the right or downward.

Exercise 1. Because your mirror image and that of an object behind you are at different distances from you, it is possible to sensitively utilize parallax to detect inaccuracies in your movement while stepping. Stand in front of a mirror and observe the reflection of yourself and that of an object behind you. Try doing the movement, "Preparation." As you shift your weight to the right, you will notice your image moving to the left relative to that of the object. Next, while you step into a shoulder width with your left foot, you should be able to detect absolutely no actual leftward movement of your head. Otherwise, you are committing your weight before the foot is touching the floor (not "stepping like a cat").

Exercise 2. Do movements of the Taiji form while viewing the reflection of the top of your head against the background. Note the extent to which your head moves up and down as you step and make transitions.

It should be noted that the perception of the size of an object is based not just on the size of its image on the retina but also how far away we estimate the object to be. To understand this fact, hold your thumb close to an eye and look at a large distant object (such as a door) through that eye. Even though your thumb may produce a larger retinal image than that of the door, you still perceive the door to be much larger than your thumb. The following example demonstrates that we correct our perception of the size of an object based on how far away we estimate the object to be.

You have probably observed that the sun seems noticeably larger when it is near the horizon than when it is overhead. When viewed through a telescope, however, the sun actually appears very slightly smaller when near the horizon—not larger. The fact that the sun only appears larger when viewed with the unaided eye suggests that the phenomenon is psychological. The explanation is that when the sun is overhead we have no way of judging its distance, but when we view the sun on the horizon we see it far behind other distant earthly objects. We know that it is much farther away than those objects, so we perceive it as larger than when it is overhead.

Experiments have been done with subjects viewing two identical spheres. One sphere was suspended overhead, and the other was moved along the horizon until both spheres appeared to be the same size. The sphere on the horizon was then measured to be farther from the subject than the one overhead.

Parallax is a dependable observational tool when stationary objects are in our field of vision and movement is on our terms. Parallax can also be useful in a self-defense situation if properly utilized in conjunction with the myriad other ways of processing information. But dependence on parallax at the expense of these other ways may be problematic. For example, it is possible to detect the initiation of a punch or kick by small movements of an opponent against a background. However, predicting when it its time to move to safety by simply looking at an opponent's body, fist, foot, etc., is really a bad idea. Our processing of such sense data by the analytical mind is much too slow for us to react in time. Also, we can be attacked by something or someone else while we look at the opponent's head, foot, or fist. Vision is only one of a number of effective ways for receiving sense data. Hearing, feeling temperature changes and air currents, and experiencing the opponent's intention to attack (intention is discussed in Ch. 4) all tend to be disregarded when vision—especially hard vision—is employed.

Hard vision is the vision most of us use most of the time. It involves "looking"—fixing on a small region of detail such as words on a page or computer screen or even a distant object such as a star. Soft vision is preferable to use in situations where we must perceive movement over a wide expanse. Soft vision involves "seeing"—comprehensively processing everything in our visual field rather than fixating on detail. The main difference between the two types of vision is in how the sense data coming in through the eyes is processed. For those able to do so, soft vision also involves diverging the axes of the eyes beyond parallel. Soft vision is an important tool when used along with all the other tools of perception.

To understand the value of practicing soft vision, it will be productive to try the following experiments,[24] which demonstrate how using soft vision affects your balance. They are listed in increasing order of improvement of your balance:

Experiment 1. Stand on one foot and look at the raised foot while moving it in different ways. Notice your balance or lack thereof. Your lack of balance demonstrates that looking at your foot makes it almost impossible to visually sense your own movement relative to your surroundings.

---

24. Repeated from Robert Chuckrow, *Tai Chi Walking*, YMAA Publication Center, Boston, MA, 2002, pp. 27–28.

Experiment 2. Stand on one foot and look at a spot on the wall or fixed object while moving the raised foot in different ways. Notice your balance or lack thereof. Your improved balance demonstrates that looking at a fixed spot (hard vision) is better than looking at your foot. But looking is not the best way to sense your own movement relative to your surroundings. Using the central field of your vision gives the most detail (unnecessary here) but is not as sensitive to movement as your peripheral vision.

Experiment 3. Stand on one foot and soften your vision while moving the raised foot in different ways. Look at nothing in particular but allow the whole panorama of your peripheral vision to permeate your awareness. Notice your balance or lack thereof. Your further improved balance demonstrates that soft vision enables you to optimally sense your own movement relative to your surroundings.

Exercise 1. Using soft vision, try doing the sections of the Taiji form requiring the most balance. Notice how the way you use your eyes is related to your balance or lack thereof. Then, become aware of the way you use your eyes in daily life.

CIRCLES IN FORM—COORDINATING CIRCULAR MOVEMENT WITH STEPPING, SHIFTING, AND TURNING

In Taiji movement, the hands do circular movement in all three planes while the body moves along straight lines and rotates about a vertical axis.[25] One exception is that of striking movements, in which the arms move along straight lines. One of the challenges of Taiji movement is coordinating the shifting and turning of the body with the circular movement of the arms and hands. For example, in "Cloud Hands," after a step to the left with the left foot, such coordination requires that the shifting of the body onto the left foot begins just after the two hands cross the horizontal diameter of the circle on which the hands are moving (see Fig. 3-3). When the hands are exactly at the horizontal diameter, they should only have a vertical component of motion. Therefore, the body should have no shifting or turning movement, which would add an unwanted horizontal component to the motion of the hands. At the part

---

25. By contrast, in Bagua movement, the hands do circular movement in all three planes while the body moves along a circle and rotates about a vertical axis, and in Xingye movement, both the body and hands move on a straight line.

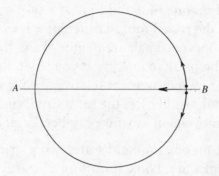

Fig. 3-3. *Line AB represents the horizontal diameter of a vertical circle on which the hands are moving in "Cloud Hands." The centers of the hands are represented as dots on the right, and their respective movements are represented by the arced arrows. Immediately after the hands pass the horizontal diameter, the body should start moving to the left (shown by the arrow on the diameter). Before the hands cross the diameter, the body should be moving to the right. Otherwise, the shifting of the body and the movement of the hands are not mutually coordinated.*

of the movement shown in Fig. 3-3, the motion of each hand is starting to have a component to the left. At this instant, the body should be starting to shift to the left in order to complement the circular motion of the hands.

   If the body shifts too early, before the hands reach the horizontal diameter, a motion shown in Fig. 3-4 occurs (the motion of the hands

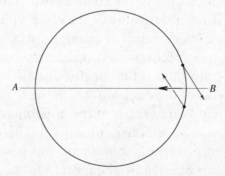

Fig. 3-4. *Line AB represents the horizontal diameter of a vertical circle on which your hands would be moving were the shifting of the body and the motion of the hands not mutually coordinated. Because the body here shifts to the left (shown by the arrow on the diameter) before the hands cross the horizontal diameter, the hands move along the diagonal straight lines shown, not on circles.*

becomes more along diagonal straight lines than on circles). If the body shifts after the hands reach the horizontal diameter, it usually means that the hands are moved independently of the motion of the body, by awkward strength.

Of course, the preceding analysis, using "Cloud Hands" as an example, applies to almost every movement of the Taiji form.

CONCAVE/CONVEX SHAPES

There are a number of regions of the body that naturally have a concave shape. Examples are: the armpit, the soft "V" just above the sternum (interclavicular notch), the "tiger's mouth" or *Hu Kou* (the webbed region between the thumb and forefinger), just above the elbow (on the back of the arm), the antecubital fossa (the depression on the inside of the elbow), the region under the jawbone, under the ribs, under the cheekbones, behind the ears, the hip joint, and the eye sockets, to name a few. These vulnerable regions of an opponent can be used to control him or as places to attack him. Certain indentations of your body such as the wrist, tiger's mouth, and instep can be used for hooking a body part of the opponent and controlling him.

Most of the above parts of the body have a shape that is impossible to change from concave to convex. However, the arms *do have* the capacity to change from concave to convex. Throughout Taiji movement, the shape of each of the inner and outer surfaces of each arm alternate between concave and convex. When the outer side of the arm is convex (yang) the inner side is concave (yin). Similarly, when the inner side is convex (yang), the outer side of the arm is concave (yin). During the movement, the leading (active) surface is usually convex, and the trailing surface is concave. This alternation is, of course, that of yang and yin, respectively, but it is much more than that. From a health and healing point of view, this convex/concave alternation involves massaging and gently stretching acupuncture meridians.

From a self-defense point of view, Sam Chin taught me that when an opponent contacts your wrist, that point of contact should feel to the opponent to be part of an impenetrable, protective sphere enclosing your body. As the opponent moves his hand to strike your body or head, a small turning movement of your body should cause the strike to slide away from its target and the opponent to lose balance. This situation is very similar to what occurs when a person hits a heavy bag off center: The bag turns on its axis, and the person slides off, losing his balance. The only difference is that the heavy bag is cylindrical, not spherical.

In order for the defense just described to work, the convexity or concavity of the surface of your arm presented to the opponent is absolutely critical in controlling him. If an arm with a surface not following the principles outlined next is presented to an opponent, it will facilitate his easy entry to the center of your body, whereas following those principles will facilitate your controlling him. Consider next the differences between presenting a concave and a convex shape to the opponent. For this discussion, convex and concave are as seen by the opponent when he contacts the *inner* surface of your arm. It is also assumed that the arm is opened sufficiently that the wrist joint is outside your shoulder joint. See Figs. 3-5 and 3-6 for convex and concave shapes, respectively, of arms.

Convex Shape. The reason for the control resulting from a convex shape is as follows: Imagine that the opponent contacts the inner surface of your right arm at a point P with his left hand. First assume that your arm presents a convex shape by extending the inside of your arm (see Fig. 3-7). Note that the perpendicular to the surface of your arm at P projects away

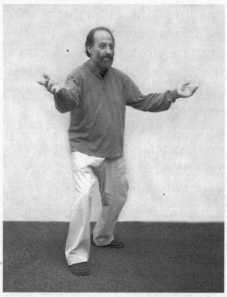

Fig. 3-5. *Convex shape of arms when wrist joints are outside of shoulder joints.*

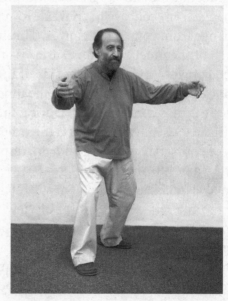

Fig. 3-6. *Concave shape of arms when wrist joints are outside of shoulder joints.*

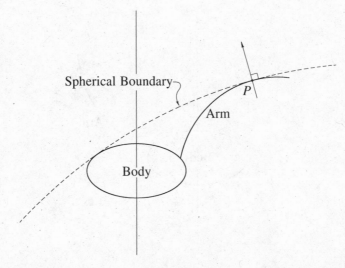

Fig. 3-7. *A schematic representation of an arm correctly used to deflect an attack. Point P is the point of contact of the opponent on the inside of your forearm. Your arm can project in the direction perpendicular to the convex surface at the point of contact. This direction is away from your body and toward the opponent. An opponent should feel as if P is a point on the surface of a spherical boundary enclosing your body. An attack to your body can then be safely deflected by turning your body counterclockwise.*

from your body, toward your opponent. Exerting a small force toward your opponent's center allows you to control his center of mass.

As far as the opponent is concerned, *P* is a point on the surface of a sphere enclosing your body. If the opponent feels that there is an opening (because, visually, your body seems unprotected), he will naturally try to attack your center. As he moves in to attack your face or body, your turning counterclockwise and continuing to project from a convex shape causes the spherical relationship to continue. Once the opponent's attack has passed your center, you can bend your elbow to change the shape of your arm from convex to concave. You then turn clockwise and control the attacker's wrist by hooking your thumb over it. Now you control the opponent, have broken his balance, are inside his space, and are able to attack him.

Concave Shape. If, instead, the opponent contacts the inner surface of an arm presenting a concave shape (see Fig. 3-8), the perpendicular to that surface at the point of contact projects away from your body and toward the opponent but much less so than for a convex shape. You can only turn

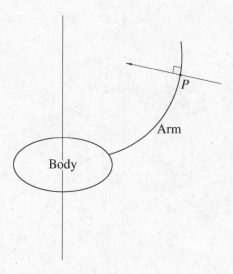

Fig. 3-8. *A schematic representation of the arms incorrectly used to deflect an attack by rotating the body. The perpendicular to your arm at the point of contact is here directed much more toward your body than in the convex case. As you turn to deflect an opponent's strike, he will be able to reach your body.*

counterclockwise to deflect the opponent's attack. As you turn, you counter his force but do not neutralize it. The (unwanted) result is bringing him toward your body, which he can easily attack.

Principle Governing Alternation of Convex and Concave Arm Shapes

When a wrist joint is between the median plane of the body and a sagittal plane[26] passing through the shoulder joint, the *outer* surface of the arm needs to present a convex shape to the opponent (with palm facing you, as in "Ward off Left"). When the wrist joint is outside the sagittal plane passing through the shoulder joint, the inner surface of the arm needs to present a convex shape to the opponent, palm facing out. It may seem that having your arm in this latter position and shape is weak and may well be perceived to be so by the opponent. However, it is actually advantageous to you; as soon as the opponent makes a move, it is felt by the sensitive surface of the inside of your arm.

---

26. Recall that a sagittal plane is any vertical plane parallel to the median plane.

INDEPENDENCE OF MOVEMENT VERSUS UNIFICATION

Our goal is to do movement through unification of body and mind; that is, each part of the body should be connected to every other part through a pervasive awareness and muscular extension. We must also be able to move parts independently. It may seem that moving parts independently is antithetical to the principle of unified motion. But in order to even know if your movement is unified, you must first be able to move all parts independently. Otherwise, how would you know if the movement is unified and exact?

Thus, at the beginning, it is important to do all movement the way the teacher shows. This manner of moving develops coordination, awareness, and the externals of Taiji movement but not correct force, which takes much longer to attain. Next, it is important to attain the ability to do movement using muscular extension rather than muscular contraction. Then the movements become coordinated through unification rather than through mere skill in moving many parts independently.

Unfortunately, many practitioners never reach the stage of doing unified movement using muscular extension but are able to refine contractive muscular action to *appear* as if the movement were correct. That is, even though a person appears to move in a unified manner, it does not mean that the movement comes from correct strength. Of course, using correct strength will naturally make movement unified. Anyone adept at doing correct movement by using muscular extension can immediately see whether someone's movement utilizes contraction or extension.

SIMULTANEITY AND "THE BIG HAND AND THE LITTLE HAND"

Often in Taiji, different parts of the body start at the same time, move different distances at different rates, but reach their destinations simultaneously (analogously to the hands of a clock). Initially, one of the most difficult tasks is to coordinate different movements of different parts of the body at different rates. Beginners must start by using their eyes, possibly a mirror, and fine-motor contractive muscular movement to attain such simultaneity. Eventually, with correct practice, the mind becomes unified with the whole body, and all movement is accomplished by using muscular extension. That is, muscular extension and its concomitant flow of qi propels, unifies, and coordinates Taiji movement.

THE IMPORTANCE OF NATURAL MOVEMENT

There are two main reasons for practicing natural movement. One reason is that you get proficient at whatever you practice, and if you practice moving unnaturally, you will get proficient at *that*. Habitual unnatural action will take its toll on your health and make you vulnerable to injury. If you practice moving naturally, you will, instead, reap health benefits and be less likely to become injured or wear out your body. The other reason for practicing natural movement is that, in a self-defense situation, unnatural movement will immediately alert your opponent and telegraph your intention. On the other hand, natural movement is much more likely to be disregarded by an opponent, giving you an advantage. Consider the following example as an illustration of natural versus unnatural movement:

Let us say that you bump into a folding chair and knock it over. It will have a characteristic way of falling and collapsing that follows the laws of physics. You may be surprised or embarrassed that you caused the chair to fall. However, nothing in the chair's behavior will evoke a response of concern that there is anything seriously wrong. If, instead of behaving according to the laws of physics, the chair spontaneously made some unnatural movement such as unfolding and then springing back to its original state and location, it is certain that you would be quite alarmed at this unnatural occurrence, and you would probably be talking about it for a long time to come.

Much Taiji movement has its roots in dealing with an opponent through actions that continuously evolve. Such a manner of moving is advantageous because it is so natural that the opponent does not react and falls behind. Any time there is a discontinuity in your movement (usually initiated by intention and contractive muscular action), it will serve to alert the opponent. The following is an anecdote that demonstrates the effectiveness of natural action in everyday life:

Before retiring from teaching high school, I was obligated to attend a yearly founders-day ceremony. My job was to take attendance and sit with my advisees during the ceremony. After having attended dozens of such ceremonies, I could not stomach one more. After taking attendance, and just before entering the assembly hall, I "suddenly realized that I had forgotten something very important." Of course, I was just acting. To retrieve the "forgotten" item, I ran in the opposite direction to that which everyone was walking. Next, I was outside the building. Then, I was on the subway train and on my way home.

The next day, I asked my advisees about the ceremony. They could not believe that I was not there and swore that I was sitting with them the entire time. It was because I behaved naturally and openly that no one had the thought that I was making an escape. I probably would have been noticed had I tried to sneak out.

TAIJI STEPPING

Stepping Like a Cat

One of the fundamental principles of Taiji is what is referred to as "Stepping like a cat," which means that, in every step, the foot must contact the ground with no discontinuity. That is, when your foot contacts the ground, there will be no sound, not even any sensation of having made contact until sufficient weight is on that foot to make you realize that the foot is down (as opposed to touching with impact, however slight).

For many practitioners, stepping by 90° or more in Taiji movement is done clumsily by using quite a bit of contractive muscular force. How is it possible to achieve effortlessness and continuity of stepping, especially with the need to take the 135° step that occurs after "Cross Hands," after "Repulse Monkey," and during and immediately after "Four Corners"?

First, the legs must be very strong so that you can sink into the rooted leg and still relax. That way, the stepping foot is closer to the ground. Second, the stepping leg—*especially the knee*—must be very relaxed and liquid during stepping. Third, your balance must be undisturbed by the stepping. This last criterion requires, among other things, that stepping be a result of muscular extension, not muscular contraction.

Stepping by Utilizing Muscular Extension Rather than Contraction

When muscular contraction is employed to lift your leg and open the hip joint, the muscles that go from your pelvis to the outside and front of your leg pull that leg. The reaction[27] to this action is that the other end of the muscle pulls your pelvis out of your rooted leg. The resulting movement is thus awkward and unbalanced. On the other hand, when muscular extension is used to lift your leg and open the hip joint, the

---

27. Action and reaction are discussed in Ch. 4.

muscles that go from your pelvis to the inside and back of your leg push that leg. The reaction to this action is that the other end of the muscle pushes your pelvis into your rooted leg. Thus, employing muscular extension in stepping makes your body more rooted and balanced.

The difference in employing muscular extension rather than contraction in 135° steps is especially noticeable. In such steps (e.g., in "Carry Tiger to Mountain"), many practitioners tend to lose shoulder width in the final posture or fail to "step like a cat." Stepping with extension is important for eliminating these problems.

The Natural Swing of the Legs During Stepping

The natural swing of the lower leg assists stepping as follows: Let us say that the left foot starts out forward of the knee, as in the posture, "White Crane Spreads Wings." As you then start to step into "Brush Knee," the hip joint of the left leg starts to open, and the left foot starts to become airborne. If the knee joint is loose, gravity causes the lower leg to swing backward to a position below the knee. But the lower leg is now moving and will continue to swing until it reaches the end of its swing an equal distance behind the knee. Then it will swing an equal distance forward of the knee, back to its original position. Coordinating the step into "Brush Knee" with the back and forth swing of the lower leg greatly assists in stepping naturally and effortlessly. The reason is that during most of the motion of the leg, the shin and foot are closer to the body than if extended all the time, and less extension requires less strength.

Let us next consider stepping from the viewpoint of yin and yang.

Yin and Yang of Stepping

Yin is passive, yielding, earthy, and supportive, whereas yang is expansive, active, upward, and outward. When your weight is all on one leg, that leg is yin (supportive, earthy, inactive, yielding), and the stepping leg is yang (active, upward, outward, expansive). To analyze the alternation of yin to yang in stepping, consider, for example, the transition from "Beginning" to "Ward off Left."

After the hands come down in "Beginning," the weight is equally distributed between both feet. Next the weight shifts 100% onto the left foot, and the body sinks and turns to the right, pivoting the right foot 90° outward. The body has now turned 45° to face northeast. If the right foot turns passively (as a result solely of the turning of the body), it will have only turned 45°, or half way. Also, there is no separation of yin and yang between the two legs because both legs will have been yin. In order for the right leg to turn twice as much as the body and for yin and yang to be balanced, the right leg must be active, which must come from extension of the inner muscles of the leg.

The correct way of executing the transition from "Beginning" to "Ward off Left" is as follows: As a small amount of weight beyond 50% goes to the left leg, that leg has become slightly more than 50% yin. Simultaneously, the right leg must become an equal amount more yang (active, outward, expansive). This change occurs not only by the decrease in weight on the right leg but also by a corresponding aliveness and outward pivoting of that leg. This action can occur correctly only by the use of muscular extension.

When the body has turned 45° and the right leg has turned 90° and is totally empty (no pressure on the ground), then the weight starts to shift onto the right foot. With every increase in weight on the right foot (and corresponding increase in yin), the left foot must experience a corresponding aliveness (and corresponding increase in yang) by means of muscular extension. So when the left foot is ready to step north, it is totally alive and ready to do so (100% yang). Stepping this way throughout the entire form will be found to be smoother, more balanced, and effortless.

By contrast, during this step with the left leg, many practitioners simply drape the left foot on the ground. Then, in stepping, the left leg suddenly transforms from totally yin to totally yang, which causes the body to lurch and the stepping to be clumsy and difficult.

A different yin/yang error frequently occurs in the transition from "Downward Single Whip" to "Golden Cock Stands on One Leg." Here it is important to get the weight off the right foot continuously rather than discontinuously as it becomes airborne. Should this transition be discontinuous, the transfer of weight to 100° on the left leg becomes clumsy and discontinuous.

---

28. The characterization *toe pivot* is inappropriate because the pivot should be done on the ball of the foot.

Heel Pivot or Ball Pivot?

In the Taiji form there are a number of places where there is a heel pivot, a ball[28] pivot, or both in succession. The question arises, what principle determines whether a ball pivot or a heel pivot should be done in a given move? There are at least two different principles involved: (1) a principle pertaining to the mechanics of movement and (2) a principle pertaining to yin and yang. These two principles are discussed next:

(1) First consider pivots of the right foot. When the right foot pivots clockwise on the ball, the center of that foot arcs inward (toward the left foot), thereby narrowing the stance. Similarly, when the right foot pivots clockwise on the heel, the center of that foot arcs outward, thereby widening the stance. Should narrowing of the stance be required, a clockwise ball pivot of the right foot suffices, and, should widening the stance be required, a clockwise heel pivot suffices. This analysis can be extended to counterclockwise rotations of the right foot and to clockwise and counterclockwise rotations of the left foot.

An example of the above principle applies to the transition just before "Separate Right Foot." As the body turns to the left, the right foot pivots counterclockwise on the heel, bringing the center of that foot closer to the left foot. Next, the right foot pivots clockwise on its ball, bringing the center of that foot even closer to the left foot. Each pivot narrows the width of the stance, which is desired. The following are more such examples:

Consider, for example, the transition into the second stance of "Fair Lady Works Shuttles." Here, some people pivot clockwise on the heel of the right foot as that foot turns out in preparation for stepping, whereas others (especially those of Zheng's lineage) pivot clockwise on the ball of that foot before the foot becomes airborne. I will make a case for Zheng's way of pivoting in terms of the principle of yin and yang:

(2) The transition of a foot from (a) fully supporting the body to (b) empty and stepping is one of yin into yang. Yin can be characterized as supportive, inactive, and earthy—a characterization that applies to a foot supporting the entire weight of the body. Yang can be characterized as active and expansive. Of course, yin must evolve into yang continuously, not abruptly. If you do the transition mentioned above Zheng's way (on the ball), I think you will find that yin transforms into yang more continuously than when the pivoting is on the heel. When the weight ebbs out of the stepping foot, its initial pivoting movement on the ball is more passive

than active, making the transition from yin to yang more continuous. By contrast, when the weight ebbs out of the stepping foot, its initial pivoting movement on the heel is initially more active than passive, making the transition from yin to yang discontinuous. Thus, Zheng's way, pivoting on the ball, is preferable.

Furthermore, in the example just discussed, when pivoting on the ball of a foot, the motion of the center of that foot is in the direction of the step, whereas the motion of the center of the foot when pivoting on the heel is not in the direction of the step. That is another reason for pivoting Zheng's way. The distinctions here are, of course, more for understanding the principles involved than for supporting my teacher's way.

As another example, if the stance in "Downward Single Whip" is not large enough, it is difficult to descend sufficiently. There are a few ways of achieving the correct length and width for this posture. The following way illustrates the principles of this section: After stepping with the left foot in the previous posture, "Single Whip," instead of pivoting the right foot inward on its heel, pivot outward on the ball. This action widens the stance. Next, in the transition into "Downward Single Whip," pivot the right foot outward on its heel as usual. Then, after shifting the weight onto the right foot, if further widening of the stance is necessary, pivot the left foot outward on its ball instead of pivoting it inward on its heel. This action further widens the stance just before descending.

BENEFITS OF PRACTICING ON UNEVEN GROUND

Until recently, I sought out the most level, even surface for practice. During the past several summers, I have held classes in a nearby park, which tends to be on a slope and have fairly uneven ground. Early on, I started to realize that every step required a unique adaptation of my foot from its accustomed level placement on a level, smooth floor to a placement that conformed to the slope and unevenness of the ground. I realized that the resulting awareness I developed was a valuable asset and made practicing outdoors more enjoyable. Instead of uneven, sloped ground being undesirable, it is an opportunity to add a dimension to your practice every now and then.

WUJI AND TAIJI IN THE FORM

According to ancient Chinese Daoist philosophy, before Taiji (yin and yang) existed, there was Wuji, the void. Wuji then separated into yin and yang. There is a parallel in Western religious teachings; namely, first there was a void, and then God created heaven and earth, day and night, and man and woman.[29]

The philosophy of the evolution of Wuji into Taiji is embodied in the initial movement, "Preparation," of the Taiji form as follows: We start with the weight evenly distributed between the two feet, heels touching, and arms hanging by our sides. This way of standing has no movement and no separation of yin and yang. As we start to move, we shift all the weight onto the right foot, sink onto the right foot, and turn to the right. At the same time, the arms become "alive" and separate slightly from the body, palms rotating to face the rear. The turning of the body helps the left foot rotate clockwise and move out a shoulder width from the right foot. Starting to move by sinking downward and activating the arms separates yin and yang in the down and up directions, respectively. Shifting all the weight to the right foot and stepping with the left foot separates yin and yang in the right and left directions, respectively. Moreover, sinking the weight and having the arms become alive separates yin and yang in the vertical direction. Thus, when you are standing with feet parallel, ready to start raising the arms in the next movement, you are in a state of Taiji.

What about separating yin and yang in the forward and backward directions? This question puzzled me for quite a while. The admonition "han xiong ba bei," which can be translated as *hollow the front, expand the back* (discussed in Chapter 5) is the key. Observing this admonition causes an accompanying activation of yin and yang in the forward and backward directions, respectively. Note that it is the lower back that expands and does so actively, using muscular extension. The front hollows passively. The distinction between passive and active movement will be treated in the beginning of the next chapter.

---

29. Note that in western culture, we tend to put the yang element first. Otherwise we would say earth and heaven, down and up, slow and fast, cold and hot, dark and light, and woman and man. The Chinese, who are aware of the tendency to put yang first, do the opposite, e.g., yin and yang, not yang and yin.

T'ai Chi comes from Wu Chi and is the mother of Yin and Yang.
—Wang Tsung-yueh[30]

After "Preparation," which expresses Wuji, the next movement, "Beginning," is really Qigong, and the movement after that, Ward off Left," is a study in peng (see the section on peng in Ch. 1). Thus, the first three movements in the empty-hand Taiji form emblemize, in order of importance, the essence of Taiji: As a philosophy, it is based on the balance of yin and yang; as a system of health, it is based on Qigong; and, as a martial art, it is based on subtle rather than brute strength. In the now-popular Beijing Twenty-Four-Movement Taijiquan Yang Form, "Ward Off Left" is replaced by "Parting the Wild Horse's Mane," which even more dramatically embodies peng.

BEING IN THE MOMENT

Recently, I was teaching a physics class, and one student said, "I didn't do well on the last test, and I am worried about my understanding of this material on the next test." I replied affectionately, "You are in both the past and the future. As a result, you are losing an opportunity to be in the present and learning the material being taught right now." By worrying about the previous test and the next test, this student was creating a state of mind that sabotaged his chances to learn right then and there. The student would have been better off devoting his energy to formulating a specific question about the current material.

Whenever we are in a situation that demands our attentiveness but our thoughts go to the future, we are then probably in the past because the present passes us by. In daily life, being in the past or future puts us at a disadvantage and can have severe consequences in a self-defense situation or when driving a car or crossing a street.

Staying in the present is very difficult for most of us. An excellent way to practice being in the moment is in doing the Taiji form. As you move, notice whether or not your attention shifts to what came before or what comes next. If you detect such a departure from your being in the moment, simply ease yourself back. As time goes by, you will find your attention shifts away less and less.

---

30. *The Essence of T'ai Chi Ch'uan, The Literary Tradition*, Edited by Benjamin Pang-jeng Lo et al., North Atlantic Books, Berkeley, CA, 1985, p. 31.

4

Dynamics of Movement

PASSIVE VERSUS ACTIVE MOVEMENT IN TAIJI

An understanding of the interplay between active and passive movement is very important to Taiji because passive movement provides many of the important benefits that many other systems of exercise and martial arts do not. Active movement occurs when the muscles that ordinarily move bones do so through contracting or extending. Passive movement occurs when part or all of the body undergoes movement—not through the muscular contraction or extension that normally would initiate that movement but through a different agent or combination of agents. Such agents include the action of gravity, the centrifugal effect of circular motion, hydraulic pressure, linear momentum, angular momentum, the elasticity (spring effect) of our bodily tissues, another person or agent moving us (as in massage or moving water), or a totally different set of muscles doing the movement. The following will clarify the above agents of passive movement:

CONCEPTS PERTAINING TO YOUR MOTION, CHANGE IN MOTION, AND EXERTION OF FORCE

We will next treat the above-mentioned agents of passive movement conceptually and then show how they produce passive movement. Some understanding of each of these agents will be required for reading some of the analyses that follow in subsequent chapters.

Inertia

Inertia refers to the tendency of an object at rest to remain at rest and of an object in motion to remain in motion at the same speed in a straight line. A consequence of inertia is that it takes an external force to initiate any change of the direction or speed of translational movement. Because non-action is one of the most basic Taiji principles, it is essential to recognize that unnecessarily interfering with or stopping motion is at a cost.

If a body is able to rotate about a fixed axis, inertia similarly applies; namely, if the body is not rotating, it will tend to remain so, and if it is rotating, it will tend to keep its same rotation. A consequence of rotational inertia is that if the body as a whole is undergoing rotational motion, in order to reduce or increase that rate of rotation, an external force must be applied (a) a distance from the axis of rotation and (b) directed perpendicular to that axis.[31]

A good example of how inertia applies to Taiji is in the transition from "Press" and "Push." As the body shifts rearward, the hands, which are in front of the body, tend to stay where they are. Thus, as the body moves rearward, the distance of the hands from the body increases. Then, as the body moves forward, the distance of the hands from the body decreases. Then, as the body again moves rearward, the distance of the hands from the body increases.

It should be noted that even in the absence of an external force, it is possible for a rotation of an arm or leg to affect the rotation of the body, as will be discussed under the section on angular momentum later in this chapter.

Newton's Third Law (Action and Reaction)

In analyses that follow in this and later chapters, the concept of action and reaction will be applied to muscular action and its internal effects.

A common statement of Newton's third law is: "For every action, there is an equal and opposite reaction." This version lacks the word *force* and, therefore, is of little use. A more scientific way of stating Newton's third law is: "If object *A* exerts a force on object *B*, then *B* exerts an equal and opposite force on *A*." Thus, if you push a door with a given force, the door exerts a force of the same magnitude back on you (see Fig. 4-1).

---

31. The component of the force perpendicular to the axis multiplied by the distance of its line of action from the axis is called *torque*.

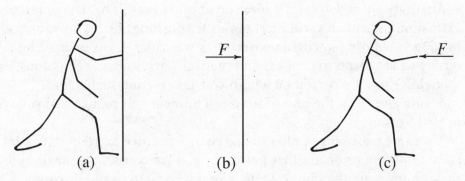

Fig. 4-1. *In part (a) of the above figure, a person is pushing a door with a force* F. *Part (b) shows the force* F *exerted by the person on the door. Part (c) shows the reaction force* F *exerted by the door on the person. A consequence of Newton's third law is that when a person exerts a force* F *on a door, the door exerts an equal and opposite force on the person.*

In order not to move backward under the action of the reaction force of the door, you will naturally push the floor backward with your feet, using friction. The reaction to the frictional force you exert backward on the floor pushes you forward and balances the force exerted by the door on you. But, if the floor were slippery (frictionless), you could not exert a backward force on it, it would not exert a forward force on you, and you would slide backward. Or, if someone unexpectedly opened the door from the other side, the force between you and door would disappear. An untrained person pushing a door that suddenly opened would likely fall forward, continuing to rely for balance on a force now absent. Falling forward would be much less likely to happen to a Taiji practitioner using correct force, as will be discussed next.

Taiji deals with interactions of people with one another, not with objects. By Newton's third law, if you exert a force on another person, that person will exert exactly the same force back on you. As with the door, if the person on whom you are exerting a force allows that force to be exerted, your body will be in balance. However, if that person suddenly gives way, unless you immediately adjust your internal forces and the forces your feet exert on the ground, you will momentarily fall forward.

If you exert force on another person by using muscular contraction, the muscles involved exert pulling forces, locking the body together and making it very hard to adjust to changes without conscious thought. But conscious thought takes too long. Thus, if a person on whom you are exerting force suddenly gives way, the inner forces will not immediately adjust, and you will fall forward.

Alternatively, if you exert a force on another person by using muscular extension, the muscles will exert opposite (pushing) forces on your body, making you more rooted. Moreover, using muscular extension has a liquid quality which adapts to changes automatically, without any conscious thought. Thus, if a person on whom you are exerting such a force suddenly gives way, the inner forces will immediately adjust, and you will *not* fall forward.

The same reasoning applies to *any* change in force exerted on you by another person or on another person by you (of course, the magnitudes of these changes are the same). Thus, it is easy to control and disrupt a person's balance if you learn to use muscular extension and are able to sense that the person you touch is using muscular contraction.

The following exercises, based on the above considerations, are valuable for (a) learning to sense if you are or somebody else is using muscular contraction (awkward force) or muscular extension (correct force) and (b) to show that root is weak when muscular contraction is used and is strong when muscular extension is used:.

Exercise 1. Player *A* stands in the "Ward Off Right" posture, and player *B* stands facing *A* in the "Push" posture (see Fig. 4-2). The hollow of *B*'s left hand centers on *A*'s left elbow, and that of her right hand centers on *A*'s left wrist. The pressure that *B* exerts on *A* is very light. After *A* achieves her best state of peng, *B* starts building up correct force but not to the point where *A* begins to replace muscular extension with muscular contraction. Suddenly, *B* releases her pressure. If *A*'s peng is correct, then her wrist may move slightly forward, but her body will remain motionless. Then *A* and *B* swap roles.

Exercise 2. Exercise 1 is repeated, but now *A* purposely uses muscular contraction instead of muscular extension. When *B* suddenly releases her pressure, *A*'s body will lurch forward. Next *A* and *B* swap roles.
These two exercises dramatically show the difference in stability between the use of the two different types of muscular action. This difference is of utmost importance in push-hands practice; namely, should one player use contractive force, the other player can release this force, which causes the first player's root to break. Zheng was well known for his softness during push-hands and his ability to execute clean and precise uproots of his partners. Examination of any of the videos of Zheng doing push-hands reveals that as soon as Zheng and his partner came into contact with each other, Zheng controlled his partner's balance. Zheng was able to sense and

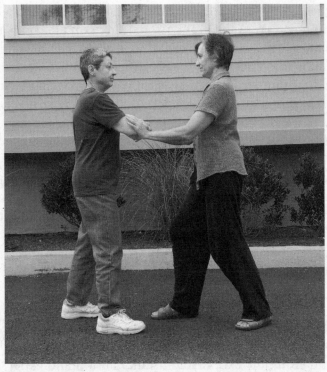

Fig. 4-2. *One student tests another for correct force. If the force is correct, the student who is in the "Push" posture can suddenly release her force, and the student in "Ward Off Right" will remain rooted.*

control even the smallest degree of contractive force in his partner. Because Zheng did not use contractive force himself, his partner had no idea that Zheng was supporting him and controlled his balance. When Zheng let up that support, his partner fell toward him visibly. Zheng then timed his push to coincide with the moment that his partner started to regain his balance.

Gravity

The gravitational force on each part of your body is constant in magnitude and direction and independent of position and motion.[32] Because the constancy of gravity makes its effect very predictable in doing movement, it would seem that in order to move, say, an arm in a natural

---

32. Actually, as an object moves away from the surface of the earth, the gravitational force on it decreases inversely as the square of its distance from the center of the earth. But even for excursions on the order of a mile above the earth's surface, this effect is much too small for a person to notice.

manner, one need only balance the gravitational effect using a constant muscular action. Whereas the gravitational force on an arm is the same whether it is hanging or held horizontally outward, the muscular action to maintain each of these positions is very different. When an arm hangs, the ligaments in the shoulder joint easily supply the force that balances gravity with no muscular action needed. But when an arm is extended horizontally, its weight and resulting leverage must be supported by muscular action. It is easy to experience that it takes the most muscular action to hold an arm out horizontally.

Therefore, as an arm lowers from the horizontal, the muscular force on it must continually decrease until it becomes zero when the arm hangs vertically. Any force beyond the minimum would violate the principle of non-action. To adjust the muscular force to be the minimum at each instant requires a constant dialogue between the brain and the muscles. Such a dialogue is an intense exercise of the nervous and perceptual system.

Professor Zheng wanted us to do "Roll Back and Press" by letting the left arm lower to the "hanging" position at one instant. I am certain that his insistence on the way of doing the movement was as a check for us to experience and eliminate excessive muscular action and experience the lack of any need for it.

Leverage

We are all familiar with the force-multiplying effects of a lever (see Fig. 4-3). If the distance between the fulcrum and the point P of application of a person's force is d_i and the distance between the fulcrum and the point of support of the rock is d_o, then the lever has a force multiplication factor (called *mechanical advantage*) of d_i/d_o. However, levers can also be used to multiply motion. A familiar example of a lever that multiplies movement is a catapult. The force that is applied on "the short end of the stick" is much greater than the projected weight, which is placed far from the fulcrum. When the large weight moves slowly through a short distance, the small weight moves quickly through a long distance, which produces the effectiveness of the catapult.

Another example of a lever that multiplies motion, called a *third-class lever*, is any limb of the human body. For example, the biceps muscle whose contraction lifts the lower arm attaches at its upper end to the bone of the upper arm and at its lower end on the bone of the lower arm very

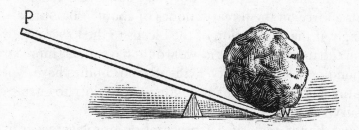

Fig. 4-3.[33]   *If the input force P is applied at point labeled P, the lever shown will multiply that force but reduce the motion of the rock by the same factor. However, if the rock at the short end of the lever is used as an input force, a smaller rock placed at P will have a correspondingly larger motion (catapult).*

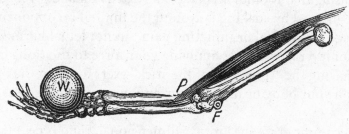

Fig. 4-4.[34]   *In the above figure, the elbow joint is the fulcrum, point P of attachment of the biceps, which applies the input force, and the output is the weight W resting in the hand. Because the input force is applied close to the fulcrum, it is much larger than W, but the motion of W is correspondingly larger than that of P.*

close to the elbow, which acts as a fulcrum (see Fig. 4-4). The result is that a small contractive movement of the biceps causes a much larger movement of the wrist. At the same time, the force exerted by the biceps on the bone of the lower arm is correspondingly larger than that of a weight lifted by the hand. For example, the distance of the application of muscular force by the biceps on the forearm is about 2 inches from the elbow joint (fulcrum). The distance of the weight in the palm of one's hand from the fulcrum is about 14 inches. Thus, motion is multiplied by a factor of about $14 \div 2 = 7$. Similarly force is divided by the same factor.

33. This figure was reproduced from Edward R. Shaw, *Physics by Experiment*, Maynard, Merrill, & Co., New York, 1897, p. 16.
34. This figure was reproduced from Edward R. Shaw, *Physics by Experiment*, Maynard, Merrill, & Co., New York, 1897, p. 28.

Thus, if a weight lifter curls a weight of 100 pounds, the tendon of his biceps exerts a force on the forearm bones of about 700 pounds!

Interestingly, if the connection of the biceps to the lower arm were further from the fulcrum than it is, we would have much more strength but correspondingly less mobility. Evidently, our bodies have evolved to have the optimal compromise of strength and mobility to enable our species to survive.

In Taiji push-hands and self-defense applications, leverage is of utmost importance in being able to control a partner or opponent using the minimum amount of force. Actually, every part of the body can become a fulcrum for the application of leverage. Studying the use of a 36-inch-long, 1-inch-diameter wooden stick for self-defense can involve much more than using that tool for striking. The extension and leverage of the stick can be utilized by snaking it around the limb of an opponent and using leverage for control or inflicting pain but not lethal harm. The proper use of leverage involves applying your force to the "long end of the stick" and having the "short end of the stick" exert force on the opponent. Any point on your body or that of your opponent can be used as a fulcrum.

A lever is commonly a one-or two-dimensional, rigid object (i.e., a straight or bent bar, respectively). How then can leverage apply to a human body, which is a three-dimensional system whose shape and rigidity vary with muscular action as a result of volition or external conditions? Because the human body is subject to psychological or external conditions, it is possible for you to cause another person's body to rigidify so that leverage can be used. The job of the Taiji practitioner is to become sensitive to the slightest wave of tension in a partner's body when it is moved away from equilibrium. Knowing how to induce that wave of tension is also an important skill.

Centrifugal Effect

When an object undergoes circular motion (such as a car rounding a curve), there is a tendency for that object to move away from the center of the circle. This tendency stems from Newton's first law, which states that an object will move at constant speed in a straight line unless acted upon by a force. Thus, in order for an object to move in a circle, there must be a force on that object, and that force is toward the center of the circle (centripetal force). In the case of a car rounding a curve, the inward force is provided by the friction of the road on the tires. However, unless there is a corresponding force on your body toward the center of the circle, your body will move in a straight line (tangent to the circle). In order for you to move in the same circular path as the car, friction, a seat belt, or door must exert a force on you toward the center of the circle in which you and the car are moving.

If you turn your body about its vertical axis, you will feel your arms start to involuntarily move outward from your body. This is the centrifugal effect of circular motion. You will also feel a hydraulic pressure in your fingers of the blood, which, by the centrifugal effect, also moves outward. Try the following exercise, called *spinning*:

Stand with both feet parallel, somewhat wider than shoulder width. Bend the knees midway between straight and totally bent. With hands on hips, turn side to side, keeping the weight centered midway between both feet. After you get the feel of rotating about a vertical axis by means of alternately bending one leg and straightening the other leg (not by twisting the trunk), let the arms go completely. Now, turning the body will cause the arms to swing and hit the body. As you increase the rotational rate, the arms will move increasingly outward and upward. This is the familiar centrifugal effect. A good example of centrifugal effect is in doing "Single Whip." As you turn to the left after "Push," both arms naturally rise and extend outward.

It should be noted that, for a given rotational rate, the centrifugal effect is proportional to the distance from the center. That is, each time the distance from the center doubles, so does the centrifugal effect. Thus, as a hand moves away from the body as a result of rotation of the body, it acts as though there were an increasing force on it away from the center of rotation. This relationship accounts for part of the whip-like effect of *fa jin*, in which a relatively small movement of the body can move a limb with speed and power. Of course, fa jin involves more than centrifugal effect; it requires the body to be completely open and unified so that force from the legs can instantly be transmitted to any part of the body. The result is that the impact of a fa-jin strike is that of the whole body, not just the striking limb.

The centrifugal effect is demonstrated dramatically by the following experiment:

Experiment: Fill a tea kettle (the kind with a wire handle) half full with cold water. Then rapidly swing the kettle over your head in an arc. Not only does the water not fall out as a result of gravity at the top of the arc, but it is pressed against the bottom of the kettle. When you do this experiment, you will feel the outward pull of the handle at the top of the arc. This demonstration works because the upward centrifugal effect at the top of the arc is greater than the downward effect of gravity.

One thing to remember is to position the spout on the trailing side of the kettle. Otherwise, when you stop the motion, water will continue to move and pour out of the spout.

Linear Momentum

In physics, *linear momentum* is defined as the product of mass and velocity. That is, the magnitude of an object's momentum is proportional to both its mass and speed. The direction of its momentum is that of its motion. If there is no external force on an object, its momentum will remain constant (conservation of linear momentum), which means that it moves at constant speed in a straight line, which is equivalent to Newton's first law.

An example of constant linear momentum is a spaceship so far from any celestial body that gravitational forces on it are negligible. The spaceship will continue to move at constant speed in a straight line. Once there is an external force on the spaceship, such as the back-pressure of the expanding gasses of its rockets, the spaceship will change its speed and/or direction.

Actually, it seems impossible to find an example where there is no force at all on a body. On earth and even hundreds of miles above the earth's surface, the force of gravity is substantial. Even the moon is held in orbit by the gravitational force of the earth. However, it is not that hard to simulate conditions of no force by reducing friction to a small value and canceling the downward force of gravity by an equal upward force. Thus, on an air-hockey table, the jets of air coming through closely spaced holes balance the force of gravity on the puck, and because the puck floats on air, friction is minimized. In that case, a puck in motion will continue to move in essentially the same direction at constant speed if no other force acts on the puck. Alternately stated, its momentum remains constant.

An application to Taiji is in push-hands. Once your partner initiates movement in any direction, he must use muscular action to change that movement. That muscular action, especially if it is contractive, can be detected by you and used to unbalance your partner.

Angular Momentum

Angular momentum, the rotational analog of linear momentum, refers to the tendency of an object in rotational motion to continue in the same motion at a constant rate. In physics, angular momentum is defined in a more complex way than for linear momentum. The magnitude of the angular momentum of an object is proportional to the product of its rate of rotation and its rotational inertia, which depends on its mass and how that mass is distributed. The farther the mass is from the center of rotation, the greater will be its rotational inertia. Thus, a ring will have a greater rotational inertia than that of a disc of the same mass and radius.

The angular momentum of an object rotating about a fixed axis will remain constant (conservation of angular linear momentum) if there is no external force having a rotational effect (called *torque*): If a force is directed through the center of the object, it will have no rotational effect. But if the force is tangential or has a tangential component, it will cause the object to slow down or speed up.

An example of constant angular momentum is a wheel rotating on an axle. If there is no friction, and no other forces have a rotational effect, the wheel will continue to rotate at a constant rate. If an applied force is directed through the axis of rotation (no external torque), the wheel will not change its rotational speed. But if the force is directed away from the axis of rotation, the wheel's speed *will* change. Consider a rotating grinding wheel after the power is removed. The force of gravity is directed through the center of the wheel and has no effect on changing its rotational speed. Were there no friction, the wheel would rotate forever. However, the friction of air and in the bearing are directed tangentially to the wheel. These forces will cause the grinding wheel to slow down and eventually stop.

One application to Taiji is in push-hands. If a push is not to a person's center, it will tend to rotate that person, making it easy for him to neutralize the push. If the push is to dead center, it will have no rotational effect and be much harder to neutralize. Similarly, if you are aware of your axis and able to change it at will, it will be very hard for a person to effect a push that you cannot neutralize by allowing it to turn you.

In an extended system, such as a spinning ice skater, her angular momentum will remain essentially constant for a short while because there is little friction of the ice and the air. When the ice skater extends her arms (making her rotational inertia increase), her rotational rate will decrease, and when she brings her arms in toward her body (making her rotational inertia decrease), her rotational rate will increase. The principle of this example comes into play in doing spirited rotational movement; namely, during the part of a turning movement when your back is turned to the opponent, bringing your arms inward increases the rotational rate, and bringing your arms outward reduces it.

Peng

Peng (refer to Chapter 1) occurs not only when arms are moving upward and outward but also when they move inward and downward. When an arm slowly lowers, there must be an upward force on it; otherwise it would fall with gravity like an inanimate object. Since, in Taiji movement, arms fall gradually, there is an upward force. If the lowering movement is done correctly (according to Taiji principles), that upward force results from muscular extension. Similarly, when an extended arm moves inward toward the body, there still must be an outward force on it resulting from peng.

Stated alternatively, Taiji movement requires balance of yin and yang at all times. Even when expanding outward when no inward force would be thought necessary, there must be a light, finely tuned inward force for balance. Similar statements apply to inward and upward actions.

Exerting a minute force in the opposite direction of motion of a limb readies the nervous system for an almost instantaneous change of direction. For example, when pushing, balancing yin and yang readies you for being pulled. The following exercise is valuable in training balance of yin and yang:

Exercise: Partners *A* and *B* face each other in harmonious 70-30 stances, wrist of the forward hand to corresponding wrist. Both partners alternate pushing and neutralizing as in one-handed push-hands. At one point, partner *A* pushes, and *B* neutralizes and, without warning, pulls *A* to the side. When pulled, *A* settles into his root. Then both partners resume doing one-handed push-hands. Then, when *B* pushes, *A* neutralizes and pulls. Both partners alternate roles in this manner for a while.

The lessons to be learned from this push/pull practice are:

1. not to over-extend your body by allowing the center of the weight distribution on your forward foot to go forward of the center of that foot,

2. how to avoid getting pulled out of your root by maintaining a readiness to move backward whenever you move forward (dot of yin in yang), and

3. settling into your rear leg to avoid losing your root when pulled.

In push-hands, once you are over-extended and pulled to the side, it is very easy for your partner to uproot you by then pushing you sideways just as your forward foot touches the ground. Be very careful in trying this sequence because it can be dangerous for the person being uprooted. In a self-defense situation, the whiplash effect of pulling an opponent with fa jin can actually result in a spinal injury.

There are other valid responses should an opponent pull you in a self-defense situation. For example, if you are pulled directly toward your opponent (not to the side), one such response is to allow yourself to be very easily pulled, so much so that you smother your opponent with an attack.

"Ratcheting"

One of the hallmarks of Zhen (Chen)-style Taiji movement and Qigong is what might be called *ratcheting*. Ratcheting, analogous to the action of a ratchet wrench (see Fig. 4-5), occurs when the movement of a limb

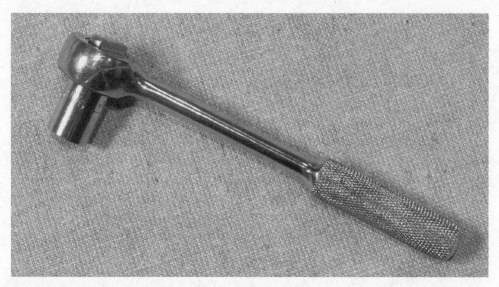

Fig. 4-5. *A ratchet wrench for tightening and loosening bolts. When the wrench reaches the end of its power stroke, to begin a new power stroke without repositioning the whole wrench, it can be turned in the opposite direction without turning the bolt.*

reaches its limit because the turning of the trunk of the body reaches *its* limit. To obtain further turning movement of that limb without moving it independently of the body, the body then turns in the opposite direction without the limb moving in space. The body then reconnects with the limb and resumes moving the limb. All throughout, peng is employed to achieve the relative movement of the body and limb.

Ratcheting has advantages beyond that in self-defense. One advantage is that of cultivating peng. Another advantage is that when the body moves during the ratcheting part of the movement, the muscles that normally move the limb relax and are moved passively. This passive movement noticeably increases the flow of qi. For this reason, certain Qigong movements utilize ratcheting.

Ratcheting is completely absent from Yang-style Taiji. Recall that Yang Lu-chan, a famous Zhen stylist, was summoned to the royal palace to teach his art to the court. Because what he knew was secret, he originated a new style, now termed *Yang style*, from which key elements were removed. Also, some elements such as very low movements, back-and-forth turning movements of the hips, and "cannon shots" were inappropriate for royalty to do.

The quiet nature of the Yang style is very appealing, but so are some of the features that are absent but remain in other styles. For this reason, some practitioners seek to learn as many styles as possible.

Hydraulic Pressure

When your arms are very relaxed, so much so that your muscles feel liquefied, you will notice changes in hydraulic pressure when you lower your arms from horizontal to a hanging position. By attaining a state wherein the muscles of your arms are in a state of muscular extension, you can feel the hydraulic pressure in your hands further increase. A similar set of conditions applies when you first sink everything into your lower abdomen, relaxing the whole trunk of the body and then energize the whole trunk of your body with muscular extension. The hydraulic pressure thus generated is easily noticed in the lower dan tian and in its contribution to peng.

When circular motion of the arms occurs, there is an additional increase in hydraulic pressure of the extremities. When the circular motion is in a vertical plane, the centrifugal and gravitational effects act together in a downward direction when the hand is at the bottom of the circle. As the arm moves toward the top of the circle, its motion usually slows, decreasing the centrifugal effect. The gravitational effect now results in hydraulic pressure being greater at the elbow. These alternations of pressure greatly enhance the flow of qi.

Another way in which hydraulic pressure works in Taiji is that, by dropping one's center of gravity at a judicious moment, the pressure at the bottom of the body can increase from its prior state. Then, this pressure "bounces" upward to initiate a movement, sometimes with power.

Kinetic Energy

In physics, energy of motion is called kinetic energy (KE). The KE of a particle is $mv^2/2$, where m is the mass of the particle and v is its speed. The KE of an extended object (as opposed to a particle) is found by adding up the kinetic energies of all of its particles. For an object that is translating and rotating at the same time, the KE is thought of as having two components, translational KE and rotational KE. In what follows, we will only be concerned with the simplest quantitative aspects of energy and will mainly treat energy qualitatively.

Work

Mechanical work is done when force is exerted on an object and there is a component of motion of that object in the direction of the force. The amount of work is equal to the force exerted multiplied by that part of the motion that is in the direction of the force. When the force is in the same direction as the motion, the work is positive, and when the force is opposite to the motion, the work is negative.

Interestingly, in the technical sense, no work is done by a stationary force or by a force directed perpendicularly to the motion of an object. So why do we get tired when exerting such forces? The answer is that, here, chemical changes are occurring in our muscles, and chemical rather than mechanical work is done.

Example 1. If you push an object along a horizontal floor at constant speed for a distance of 2 feet by exerting a constant horizontal force of 10 pounds, you will have done an amount of work equal to $10 \times 2 = 20$ foot pounds. The fact that the speed was constant during the motion means that there must be a force equal and opposite to your push, which, in this case is friction between the floor and the object. The frictional force, therefore, must be 10 pounds, directed opposite to the motion. Thus, friction will have done an amount of work equal to $10 \times (-2) = -20$ foot pounds.

Example 2. If you lift an object that weighs 10 pounds a vertical distance of 2 feet at constant speed (by exerting an upward force of 10 pounds, just balancing the force of gravity on the object), you will have done an amount of work equal to $10 \times 2 = 20$ foot pounds. During the downward motion, the force of gravity, which is exerted downward (opposite to the motion), will have done an amount of work equal to $10 \times (-2) = -20$ foot pounds. Similarly, if you lower an object that weighs 10 pounds a vertical distance of 2 feet at constant speed (again just balancing the force of gravity on the object with an upward force of 10 pounds), you will have done an amount of (negative) work equal to $10 \times (-2) = -20$ foot pounds. At the same time, the force of gravity, which is exerted downward (in the direction of the motion), will have done an amount of (positive) work equal to $10 \times 2 = 20$ foot pounds.

Potential Energy

The concept of potential energy (PE) of a mechanical system can be understood by considering the difference between examples 1 and 2, above: In example 1, you did work on the object by moving it against friction. The energy you expended then became thermal energy, which caused the object and its surroundings to rise in temperature a small but measurable amount. There is no way that the thermal energy can sponta-neously convert back into mechanical energy (we never see liquid water spontaneously converting its thermal energy to potential energy by jumping to the ceiling and becoming ice!). However, in example 2, the work that you did in raising the weight against gravity *is* readily retriev-able. All that you need to do is release the weight after lifting it, and it will fall under the action of gravity. The energy that you originally imparted to the weight now reappears as kinetic energy. It can be seen that doing work against friction is very different from doing work against gravity. In the frictional case, the energy is not immediately retrievable, but in the gravi-tational case it is. Thus, we say that when energy is expended by lifting an object against gravity, that energy is "potentially" available because it can be retrieved at a moment's notice. We, therefore, characterize the energy of position in a gravitational field as *gravitational potential energy*. Other forms of PE include electrical and spring energy. Spring PE (discussed next) is energy that can be stored in a stretched or compressed spring.

Spring Energy

Both muscles and tendons (tendons connect muscles to bones) have elasticity. Elasticity is a property of a material that enables it to recover its initial configuration when stretched or compressed. When any elastic body such as a spring is either stretched or compressed a small amount, the applied force increases proportionately to the amount by which the length of the spring is displaced from its equilibrium length (this principle is called *Hooke's law*). The reaction to the applied force is called *the restoring force*.

Spring energy comes into Taiji movement as follows: The tissues of our bodies have a spring-like effect, which means that when our tissues are stretched or compressed, they provide a restoring force that can be employed to propel a specific movement. For example, each movement of the Taiji form involves "winding up" each hand in one direction and allowing it to rotate back to the neutral position. Then the action is repeated in the opposite direction. These rotations have both a health and self-defense value.

The health benefit occurs when a wrist is gently rotated from the neutral position and then allowed to rotate back passively, under the action of the spring effect of the muscles in the forearm. It is essential to recognize the lack of need to *make* the wrist rotate back. Such movement causes the acupuncture meridians to be gently stretched and massaged, resulting in a noticeable increase in the qi benefits of doing the form.

From a self-defense standpoint, each rotation of the forearm has an effect similar to that of the rollers on which goods are sent into a supermarket from a delivery truck. When an opponent contacts your arm, its rotation causes the opponent's strike to safely roll away from your body and causes a disruption of the opponent's balance. Such a defense requires the rotations to be done naturally and coordinated with the opponent's movement.

The following exercise is designed to help you recognize the spring effect of bodily tissues.

Exercise. Stand with an arm outstretched horizontally in front of you. Try to relax as much as possible and let the arm attain its most centered alignment rotation-wise. Next rotate the hand in one direction away from the neutral orientation using muscular extension on the side that is getting longer. You should feel the restoring force increase as you rotate more. When you feel that turning further would produce too much tension, slowly release and let the hand rotate, *on its own*, back to the neutral orientation. Next repeat the exercise in the other direction. Slowly lower the arm, feeling every change as you do so. Then compare the amount of blood and qi circulation between the two hands. The hand you used for the exercise should be substantially more energized.

Many Taiji movements involve stretching of muscle tissue on the front or back of the region around the hip joints (*kua*). When a hip joint opens from its centered position, the muscle tissue in front of the body is stretched. Similarly, when a kua closes, the muscle tissue in back of the body is stretched. In the interests of simplicity, we will say here that when the kua closes, it compresses the tissues on the inside even if it is probably the case that the spring effect occurs as a result of stretching of tissues on the outside.

A good example of a movement initiated by spring energy is the transition from "Push" to "Single Whip." This transition involves turning the body 90° to the left with the weight 100% on the left leg. Here, the right foot ends up turned inward 45° from parallel to the left foot. Next, when the weight shifts to the right and the body turns to the right, the right hip joint closes, causing a compression of the tissues in the right hip joint. When this compression is released, with weight 100% on the right foot, the trunk of the body will automatically turn to the left, which is exactly the action required in stepping out with the left foot. A similar transition occurs in "Fair Lady Works Shuttles."

Moving by means of compressing a hip joint occurs in the transition from "Separate Left Foot" to "Pivot on Right Heel and Kick." In this transition, the body first turns to the right and then undergoes a 135° counterclockwise rotation, the initiation of which originates from a compression of the right hip joint.

It should be noted that receiving an opponent's energy is based on the spring effect of bodily tissues. When an opponent exerts force on you, your leg muscles experience a stretch greater than that resulting from the weight of your own body. That spring energy can be returned as kinetic energy to the attacker with devastating effect.

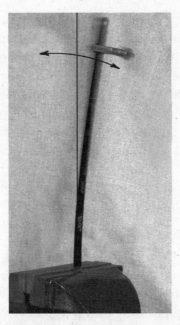

Fig. 4-6. *A vibrating hacksaw blade, one end of which is tightly held in a vise, with a small clamp attached near its free end to provide additional mass. The arced arrows indicate the direction of to-and-fro motion about the vertical axis shown.*

Periodic Motion

There is an important domain of physics that deals with periodic motion. A periodic motion is a repetitive, back-and-forth motion of an object such as a pendulum or a system consisting of a mass attached to a spring.

Two characteristics must be present for periodic motion to occur: an inertial property and an elastic property. The inertial property refers to the mass of the system and its distribution. The elastic property refers to the presence of a restoring force that causes the system to resume its original configuration when displaced from equilibrium. All physical systems vibrate at rates that depend on their elastic and inertial properties.

How the distribution and amount of mass affects vibrational frequency is illustrated by a hacksaw blade one end of which is clamped in a vise and the other end of which has an attached weight (see Fig. 4-6). The farther the weight is placed from the clamped end of the blade, the lower the natural frequency, and other factors being the same, the heavier the attached weight, the lower the frequency.

A pendulum is another system that can undergo natural vibration. A familiar example of a pendulum is a child on a swing. Because our arms and legs are like pendulums, they are also capable of periodic motion when we relax enough to permit such motion to occur. In order to build up the amplitude[35] of the vibration of a child on a swing, another person must push the child at the same frequency as that of the natural vibration and at just the right part of the swing. When it comes to our own bodies, it is possible to augment the natural swing of our arms and legs by feeding energy into that motion with the right timing. In fact, cultivating this very motion is of crucial importance in Taiji movement, and this concept will, therefore, be discussed next.

Forced Vibration

Consider a child sitting on a swing. If another person repetitively pushes the swing, a large amplitude motion builds up. However, the timing of each push is critical. If the timing and frequency are correct, the amplitude of the child's motion will increase, but if the timing and/or frequency is off, the amplitude of motion will decrease.

Exercise 1. Lightly grasp a yardstick (or similar piece of wood) with the tips of your thumb and forefinger near its end. Allow it to hang and act as a pendulum. First ascertain the natural frequency of the yardstick by displacing it to the side and letting it swing to and fro without interfering with its natural motion. Next, move your hand back and forth. First move very slowly. The yardstick will follow the motion of your hand but not have much vibration. Next, move very fast. The yardstick will again follow the motion of your hand but not have much vibration. Finally, find the frequency and timing with which to move your hand so that the yardstick has the maximum amplitude of vibration. That frequency will be the natural frequency.

Conclusion: *A system will have its maximum amplitude of vibration when forced to vibrate at its natural frequency.*

The human body can be thought of as a mechanical system whose arms and legs can swing and, if allowed to do so without restriction, have a natural frequency. In doing natural movement, an awareness of the natural frequency of arms and legs should be cultivated. Movement is maximized when the timing of movements takes such natural rates into account. The

---

35. The amplitude of a periodic motion is the maximum distance from equilibrium.

following exercise illustrates how to utilize the natural swing of your arms when doing Taiji movement and helps you find the proper timing of the turning of your body to maximize the transfer of that energy to your arms:

Exercise 2. Let one of your arms hang by your side (in place of a yard-stick). Have someone test the degree to which your arm and shoulder are relaxed by pulling your arm forward a small amount and then releasing it. Your arm should swing back and forth quite a few times with gradually decreasing amplitude.

Next, without any assistance, turn your body slightly left and right about a vertical axis. Note that even though you are rotating your body horizontally, you must confine the movement of your arm to occur in a forward vertical plane without otherwise interfering with it. Experiment with the relationship between the movement of your body and that of your hanging arm when there is a maximum transfer of energy, evidenced by attaining a large amplitude of swing. Note that at maximum transfer, the frequency of the motion of your body (*driving frequency*) and the natural frequency of your arm are the same. Note also that your body is at the end of its motion in one direction before your arm is at the end of its motion. That is, the motion of your body is ahead of the motion of your arm (actually by one-quarter of a cycle).

Next, see what happens when you rotate your body at a higher or lower frequency than the natural frequency of your arm. You should observe that the amplitude will be noticeably smaller to the extent that the *driving* frequency differs from the natural frequency.

In every step in the form (or in daily life for that matter), coordinating the movement of the body with the natural frequency of the swing of the stepping leg adds a dimension of relaxation and exuberance.

Exercise 3. This exercise is essentially the same as that suggested in the section, "Centrifugal Effect," in this chapter. Stand with both feet parallel, somewhat wider than shoulder width. Bend the knees midway between straight and totally bent. With hands on hips, turn side to side, keeping the weight centered midway between both feet. After you get the feel of rotating about a vertical axis by means of a piston-like motion of the legs (not by twisting the trunk), let the arms go completely. Now, turning the body will cause the arms to swing and hit the body. As you vary the rotational rate, note the degree to which rotational energy is transferred to your arms. The accompanying feeling of maximizing the transfer of energy is similar to that of swinging a sledge hammer.

Once you have an understanding of this principle on a physical level, it can also be applied to the motion of your partner during push-hands to achieve the maximum effect when breaking his/her root and pushing. On the higher levels, an internal movement is caused by turning the trunk of the body in such a manner that a strike is executed by a whip-like action. Such a way of striking is called *fa jin*. The advantage of fa jin is that until the strike hits, the body is relaxed and appears natural, a condition that does not telegraph the action to the opponent.

Wave Motion

Waves are a special mode of transferring mechanical energy from one region to another. In wave motion, the particles of the medium in which waves propagate undergo vibrational motion of relatively small amplitude, but the energy of that vibration propagates through relatively large distances as waves. For example, the heights of water waves are typically several inches to several feet, which means that the particles of water undergo motion of that amplitude. However, water waves can propagate for many miles. Similarly, sound waves in air can travel large distances, but the molecules of air in a sound wave undergo microscopically small vibrational amplitudes.

In Taiji, wave motion occurs microscopically as a result of vibration on the cellular level (qi) and on a gross level involving the whole body as a liquid. For either of these modalities to occur, the body must be totally devoid of contractive muscular tension and be unified through muscular extension. The result is an ability to transmit a large external force as a result of a relatively small, hidden movement.

The basic element of wave motion is the pulse, which is a short-lived disturbance of a medium that propagates it. Consider Figure 4-7, which shows four images of a long tube filled with air at atmospheric pressure, a tightly fitting, moveable piston at the left end, and a hand that can move the piston. When the piston is sharply moved a small distance to the right, the air just to the right of the piston must move with it. The air further down the tube has inertia, and tends not to move. Therefore at that instant, the air next to the piston becomes compressed, but the rest of the air in the tube remains at atmospheric pressure. Because the pressure just to the right of the piston is higher than that of the air in the rest of the tube, the air under higher pressure starts to expand to the right, thereby compressing the next region, which next expands to the right, and so on.

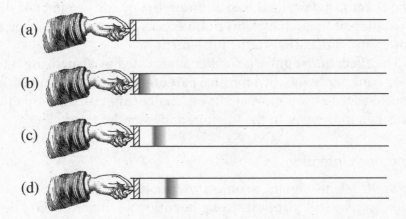

Fig. 4-7.[36] *The above figure shows a succession of events involving a long tube filled with air, a tightly fitting, moveable piston at the left end, and a hand that can move the piston. In (a), the piston rests at the end of the tube. In (b) the hand moves the piston sharply a small distance to the right and stops, compressing the air just to the right of the piston. In (c) and (d) the compression moves off to the right at the speed of sound in air. The compressed region of the air is indicated by the density of the shading in that region.*

Thus, the disturbance moves off to the right. Such a phenomenon is called a *compressional pulse*.

Note that air molecules in each part of the tube move only a short distance, whereas the disturbance can move the length of the tube, however long it is.

When the compression reaches a fixed (walled-off) end of the tube, the rigidity of the region to the right of the compression prohibits any further expansion in that direction. The only way the compression can now expand is to the left. Thus, the compression moves off to the left (is reflected).

The connection of this discussion to Taiji movement presumes that your body is in a liquefied state (song): When your body shifts to the rear, sinking your weight, the momentum of your tissues causes an inner, backward movement beyond that from shifting infinitely slowly. The result is a compression in the dan tian and rear foot. This compression then rises up through the body as a pulse that can be felt in the lower back, then up along the spine, and transmitted to the shoulders and arms. If you coordinate the subsequent forward motion of your body with this inner movement, these two movements augment each other.

---

36. The hand in this figure was reproduced from Edward R. Shaw, *Physics by Experiment*, Maynard, Merrill, & Co., New York, 1897, p. 216.

The effect just described is in addition to any spring effect of the stretching of the tissues. This pulse acts as an internal massage and adds power and unification to the movement.

The effect of the pulse is further augmented by visualizing it to move away from the body when the final part of the posture is attained. The Taiji double-edged-sword movements especially emphasize sending the extended movement to the treetops and even the stars.

Another's Intention

In a self-defense situation, unless your opponent is highly trained in Taijiquan, he will manifest strong intention a moment before he attacks. If you watch for his attack using just your eyes, you will only be able to initiate your defense after he starts to move and you have processed the associated sense data using the analytical part of your brain. However, if you use all of your senses including those yet unnamed, you will sense the opponent's intention *before* he starts to move. In fact, with training, your movement will actually occur almost involuntarily, in just the right amount, and at the right time. This way of moving is quite different from initiating movement yourself, using your eyes and analytical mind.

> It is said "if others don't move, I don't move.
> If others move slightly, I move first."
>
> —Wu Yu-hsiang[37]

The following is an exercise for sensing another's intention.

Exercise. Player *A* stands relaxed, in a feet-parallel posture, and player *B* stands behind *A*. *B* imagines attacking *A*, but she does not actually do so. If *B* holds a model knife near *A*'s back, this will facilitate sending "negative energy" to him. At first, *B* dwells in a state of non-intention, but, at a certain moment starts to "send" to *A*. When *A* senses *B*'s energy, he moves. Next *A* and *B* swap roles.

In doing this exercise with a beginner, it will become obvious that as soon as the negative energy starts, the beginner will involuntarily move slightly without realizing it.

After some training, it is good for *B* to actually attack (being careful not to do any physical harm) so that the other person can practice moving

---

37. *The Essence of T'ai-Chi Ch'uan, The Literary Tradition*, Edited by Benjamin Pang-jeng Lo, North Atlantic Books, Berkeley, CA, 1985, p. 57.

away with just the right timing. If the movement response is lacking or ill timed, *A* merely gets gently poked with a dull, wooden knife.

The feeling you get when someone attacks with intention from behind is one of urgency to move away from the danger. Developing a high degree of this feeling and an appropriate response to it will render a person well protected from harm. However, this skill will not work against an attacker who manifests non-intention.

CHANGES OF ONE TYPE OF MECHANICAL ENERGY INTO ANOTHER IN TAIJI MOVEMENTS

When energy is stored as potential energy of any type, it can be converted into kinetic energy. For example, if a mass is lifted from ground level to the top of a building, its potential energy now will have increased by the amount of work required to lift it to that height. If the mass is then allowed to fall back to the ground, its potential energy at the top will have been converted to an equal amount of kinetic energy just before it hits the ground. Similarly, if a mass suspended by a string (pendulum) is displaced from its equilibrium position (arbitrarily assumed to be at zero PE) to a given height (maximum PE) and then released, when it reaches its lowest position, its potential energy will have been converted to kinetic energy. That kinetic energy, in turn, can be spontaneously converted back into the same amount of potential energy, which means that, in the absence of any friction, the pendulum will come up to the same height on the other side (see Fig. 4-8).

One application of the above analysis is in sensing the natural swing of legs during stepping and allowing that swing to move your legs with minimal effort. Whenever the foot is rearward of the knee and that leg is lifted, if you allow the shin to swing freely, the foot will swing forward an equal distance without any effort. A similar statement applies to the upper leg; namely, whenever the thigh is rearward of the hip joint and that leg is lifted, if you allow the thigh to swing freely, the leg will swing forward an equal distance without any effort. Both of these conditions occur in "Step forward, Parry, and Punch" just after the crescent step.

Similarly, whenever the foot is forward of the knee and that leg is lifted, if you allow the shin to swing freely, the foot will swing backward an equal distance without any effort. After swinging backward, the shin will return

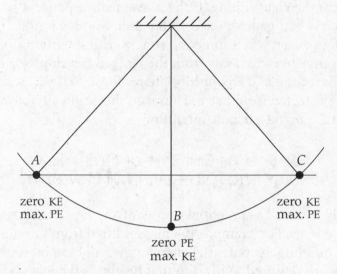

Fig. 4-8. *The above figure shows a pendulum, which consists of a mass on the end of a string fixed at its other end. When the pendulum is lifted to position A, it has its maximum PE and zero KE. When the pendulum is released, it has maximum KE and zero PE at point B. Then, when it swings to point C, it again has maximum PE and zero KE.*

to its initial angle forward of the knee. Such conditions occur in "Single Whip" during the final step with the left leg.

Allowing the leg to swing freely greatly assists in having the stepping be natural. Moreover, every step in the form (and in daily life) can become more effortless by allowing the legs to swing naturally.

The following is a somewhat different application of one type of mechanical energy changing into another: When the body lowers by giving in to gravity, it stretches the leg muscles and stores energy that can be later released. Of course, the body must be totally free of contractive muscular action, and the leg muscles must be so strong that they are able to be stretched to their limit without needing to protect themselves by contracting. Zheng Manqing wrote about this concept.[38]

The next stage is for an opponent's force on you to stretch the leg muscles beyond what the weight of your body could ever do. This is called "borrowing your opponent's energy" or "receiving energy."[39] If this stored energy is released with just the right timing, it has an amazingly powerful effect.

---

38. Cheng Man-ch'ing, *T'ai Chi Ch'uan: A Simplified Method of Calisthenics for Health & Self Defense*, North Atlantic Books, Berkeley, CA, 1981, pp. 13–16.
39. Ibid, pp. 124-125.

"Store up the jin like drawing a bow; release the jin like releasing an arrow."
—Wu Yu-hsiang[40]

Such a way of interacting has nothing to do with contracting muscles. Everything in the empty-hand Taiji form is for weeding out the use of contractive muscular action. That is why we rely as much as possible on gravity, momentum, angular momentum, spring energy, peng (extensive muscular action), etc., to do the movements. It is doubtful that anyone could perfect receiving energy just by doing push-hands, without practicing the empty-hand form. Doing the form is necessary but not sufficient; the form must be practiced correctly.

SHIFTING OF WEIGHT

In the Taiji movements, there is a repetitive shifting of the weight from one leg to the other. Sometimes the weight shift ends with 70% of the weight on the forward leg and 30% on the rear leg (e.g., "Single Whip"), and at other times, the distribution is 100% of the weight on one leg. The 100% distribution occurs during stepping and in final postures where all the weight is on the rear foot (e.g., "Hands Playing the Pipa"). It also occurs during transitions involving shifting backward and forward (e.g., "Withdraw and push"). The manner in which the shifting is produced is of utmost importance, and shifting forward has a different dynamic than shifting backward.

Shifting Backward

In shifting backward (yin action), the body releases and allows the center of gravity to descend slightly. This action is analogous to the way something might slide frictionlessly down a very slight incline. Note that shifting backward by pushing off the forward leg would be a yang action and, therefore, wrong. In push-hands practice, your partner's push moves you backward, and it is important to practice allowing the joints of the lower body to be so loose that it takes minimal force to move you backward. Similarly, in practicing the Taiji empty-hand form, it is of value to simulate the push-hands way of shifting by having gravity rather than your partner move you backward.

---

40. *The Essence of T'ai-Chi Ch'uan, The Literary Tradition*, Edited by Benjamin Pang-jeng Lo, North Atlantic Books, Berkeley, CA, 1985, p. 53.

Shifting Forward

In shifting forward (yang action), the weight is on the rear leg, and the quadriceps[41] of that leg is devoid of any contraction and stretched by the entire weight of the body and leverage. The force that propels the body forward is extension of the muscles on the back of the rear leg. To convince yourself that this way of shifting forward is correct, consider that the only other way of shifting forward is to contract the quadriceps of the rear leg, which is the use of awkward force and, therefore incorrect.

Yin and Yang in Shifting Forward and Backward

Shifting backward is a yin action. The dot of yang in this action is that the muscles on the back of the rear leg extend ever so slightly and are ready to move the body forward. Shifting forward is a yang action. The dot of yin in this action is that the muscles on the back of the front leg extend ever so slightly and are ready to halt the forward motion. This interplay of yin and yang ensures that the movement can be changed at a moment's notice to meet external conditions. One of my teachers, Sam Chin, referred to this state of readiness as "always having the motor running."

> The form is like that of a falcon about to seize a rabbit, and the shen [spirit] is like that of a cat about to catch a rat.

> —Wang Tsung-yueh[42]

TURNING OF THE BODY

There are a number of correct ways that the body turns: (1) as a result of muscular extension, (2) as a result of spring energy, (3) as a result of linear momentum being converted into angular momentum, and (4) as a result of gravity. Various combinations of these four ways can be employed to facilitate natural movement.

Turning by using muscular extension means that the muscles joining the bones of the legs to each other and the thigh bone to the pelvis extend rather than contract to cause the turning motion.

Turning by using spring action means that the natural tone of muscles and other bodily tissues when they depart from their relaxed length cause a force that can rotate (or translate) the body. Such an action can result

---

41. The quadriceps is so-called because it is a muscle that has four heads.
42. *The Essence of T'ai Chi Ch'uan, The Literary Tradition*, Edited by Benjamin Pang-jeng Lo et al., North Atlantic Books, Berkeley, CA, 1985, p. 59.

from compression or tension. An example of movement originating from spring compression occurs in the turning of the body in "Single Whip" just before the final step with the left leg. An example of movement that originates from spring tension occurs just before the turning of the body in "Turn to Sweep the Lotus." Just before that turn, the right hip joint is very open (almost 90°), causing tension in the muscles controlling that joint. A release of that tension can result in a sufficient rotational effect for that movement. Other examples occur in many places in the form.

The concept of turning by converting linear momentum into angular momentum can be understood by imagining a rod in outer space (no gravity) translating to the right. When the end of the rod hits and becomes fixed to the support, the linear motion becomes rotational motion about the point of fixing (see Fig. 4-9).[43] Such a conversion of linear motion into turning motion occurs in doing "Brush Knee." In doing "Brush Knee," the left foot steps into what will become a 70-30 stance, and the weight shifts onto the left foot until just before the left knee goes beyond a vertical line through the toes. At that point, linear motion of the body stops and is transformed into a counter clockwise rotation of the body about the left hip joint.

Turning as a result of gravity is possible by lowering the center of gravity slightly and creating an internal state in which the only way that the body can descend is if it also rotates about a vertical axis as it descends. In physics, such a limitation imposed on movement is called a

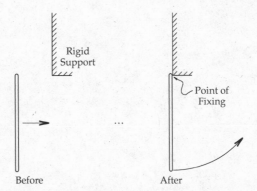

Fig. 4-9. *Before and after sketches of a rod in outer space translating to the right. When the end of the rod hits and becomes fixed to the support, the linear motion becomes rotational motion about the point of fixing.*

43. The calculation of the final angular velocity of such a rod of known length and mass in terms of its initial velocity is done in many college physics classes. In fact, my AP Physics students at Fieldston were able to do this problem.

constraint. A good example of rotation of the body occurring from gravity is the turning of the body to the left as one sits back on the left leg in "Roll Back." After the body shifts backward onto the left leg, its tendency is actually to turn to the right about the left hip joint. For the body to turn in the opposite direction (to the left), another action must come into play. One way is to simply lower the body slightly. Another way is to use the weight and momentum of the left arm, as it drops, to help turn the body to the left.

5

Seemingly Paradoxical Admonitions

Traditional Taiji Teachings are replete with admonitions, which on the surface might seem obvious, trivial, ridiculous, meaningless, or self-contradictory. Actually, these admonitions are meant to have a deeper, hidden meaning that the practitioner is expected to eventually penetrate. The following are a few such admonitions:

"ALWAYS ...," "NEVER ..."

At one time or another, teachers in all disciplines will tell students that certain actions are totally prohibited. However, the word *never* is subject to interpretation. Let us say that a mother tells her young child to stay on the sidewalk at all times and never set foot in the gutter without an adult supervising. What if a car comes onto the sidewalk? Should the child not jump out of the way in order to save his life? Also, eventually, it will be appropriate for the child to cross on his own. The principle here is: *Never* really means *first abstain from doing the action in question until you understand its problems or dangers; then use your judgment.*

"DO NOT LIFT THE SHOULDERS"

This admonition is given because rank beginners incorrectly tend to lift their shoulders. The shoulders of most people untrained in Taiji tend to be highly susceptible to sympathetic muscular tension. Unnecessarily lifting the shoulders wastes energy, restricts the mobility of the arms, telegraphs intention to an opponent in a self-defense situation, and makes the shoulders susceptible to becoming locked by an opponent. The other extreme is actively pulling shoulders downward to prevent any lifting. Therefore, it is essential that beginners develop an awareness of shoulder-lifting and work on releasing shoulders totally.

When taken literally, the admonition not to lift the shoulders is contradictory to "When one part of the body moves, all parts move; when one part is still, all parts are still." When any part of the body is totally inactive, it violates the principle that nothing should be all yin (or yang). As practitioners become more advanced, they naturally develop a looseness to the shoulders, involving minor, subtle, natural movements instead of their shoulders being totally inactive (all yin) or pulled down (all yang).

"Let the Elbows Droop"

Beginners tend to lift their elbows, sometimes as high as their shoulders, and they do so for no apparent reason. Therefore, beginners are told to let their elbows droop. Actually, advanced practitioners' elbows are usually much higher than those of beginners who pay heed to this admonition and droop their elbows downward. The reason for this discrepancy is that advanced practitioners expand their arms outward (peng). However, an elbow can only move in an arc about the shoulder joint. Thus, in order to move an arm outward, the elbow must also arc upward, and this latter motion occurs passively. Of course the outward expansion must result from muscular extension, not muscular contraction.

A long-term practitioner who doggedly follows admonitions given to rank beginners is like the dog that required treatment by an animal psychoanalyst. Unfortunately, the therapy could not be undertaken because the dog had been trained to stay off the couch.

"Taiji Movement is Characterized by Non-Intention"

Intention involves a mental decision to attain a particular goal. Non-intention involves no fixation of purpose, with a readiness to change course appropriately at a moment's notice. The ability to attain a state of non-intention is extremely important in daily life, Taiji practice, and the application of Taiji as a martial art.

In daily life, having an intention to do a particular action can result in fixating your attention and disregarding the need to change course. In driving an automobile, it can cause an accident. The following example is from a web site[44] for students who are preparing for the S.A.T. math examination: "Don't go into every question searching for a shortcut; it might end up taking longer than the normal route. Instead of seeking out math shortcuts, you should simply be mindful of the possibility that one might exist. If you go into each question knowing there could be a shortcut and keep your mind open as you think about the question, you will find the shortcuts you need."

In a self-defense situation, having an intention to do an action will immediately alert a trained opponent, who will have gained a substantial advantage. Your opponent will know that you intend to do something and may even know what you are going to do and how and when you will do it. Instead, acting without intention against an opponent who acts with intention gives *you* the advantage.

> *The opponent does not know me, but I know the opponent.*
> —Wang Zong-yue[45]

On the other hand, never having any intention is like taking non-action to an extreme—either extreme will lead to getting little if anything done. There are times when intention is necessary, even in a self-defense situation. For example, in a self-defense situation, once you become aware of an opening and initiate an appropriate attack, you must have *total* intention at the instant your punch or kick makes impact, otherwise your attack will have little effect.

Also, during an encounter with someone who wants to physically harm you, attaining a state of intention to do a false attack while initiating another attack, done without intention, will deceive that person and give *you* the advantage. For example, having an intention to throw imaginary sand in the face of an attacker might give you enough time to run away. This deception is not the same as feinting or faking, in which there is no intention to do the false action.

During self-defense practice, intention during an attack is needed to simulate a real situation in which the opponent *will* have intention to

44. *http://www.sparknotes.com/testprep/books/sat2/math2c/chapter3section3.rhtml.*
45. Yang, Jwing-Ming, *Tai Chi Secrets of the Ancient Masters*, YMAA Publication Center, Boston, MA, 1999, p. 17.

injure you. Therefore, during early stages of practice, it is often important to initiate an attack *with* an intention to harm your partner but, of course, not actually do any harm. If you attack without intention, your partner will know that there is no threat and feel no need to take any action. Practicing without intention is unrealistic and has little self-defense value. After players become more advanced, it is of value to reduce intention for the reasons already mentioned.

Therefore, we ultimately need to command a range from complete non-intention to strong intention. Acting with intention is easy, but acting without it is not, so achieving a state of non-intention requires training and sustained practice. Thus, the beginner must learn to shed intention when doing Taiji form, push-hands, and sparring but move with intention during choreographed practice of self-defense applications such as occur in the two-person form.

Here is an interesting exercise for practicing intention: If you have the opportunity to walk in a fairly crowded place such as a mall or a sidewalk in a large city, try the following: When you see someone coming in the opposite direction who will easily miss you in passing, without changing anything external to yourself, just imagine that you are going to start moving toward that person but without actually doing so. Almost always, the passerby will respond by departing from a straight-line path and moving farther away from you. Then try walking naturally without such an intention. The passerby will simply walk by without changing direction.

Or, you can try imagining your body to have enormous girth, so much so that the passerby will feel the need to move away to avoid hitting you. Note the passerby's response to your mental projection.

In self-defense, "projecting" an image of your head to be shifted from where it really is can cause your opponent's punch to miss. Similarly, projecting an image of your head to be larger than it really is can cause your opponent to punch there and not another part of your body. Moreover, projecting an image of your body to be closer than it really is will cause your opponent to punch or kick at too large a distance and miss. Knowing beforehand where and when the opponent will attack gives you an advantage.

If the opponent raises up, I seem taller; if he sinks down, I seem lower; advancing, the distance seems incredibly longer; retreating, the distance seems exasperatingly short.

—Wang Zong-yue[46]

Note that intention differs from preconception. Intention is a state of mental determination, whereas preconception involves a fixation on an idea or a particular method of achieving something (such as using a particular technique) before the opportunity even arises and by contriving things to happen according to a planned outcome.

"THE HANDS DON'T MOVE," THE "BEAUTEOUS HAND," AND "THE HAND IS NOT A HAND"

The expression, "In Taiji, the hands don't move," can be interpreted that, whereas the hands are moving in space, they barely move relative to the body; that is, the hands do not move on their own but through unification with the whole body. The beauteous hand, a concept Zheng Manqing espoused, means having the wrist and the fingers of the hand in the most neutral and relaxed alignment, which is the most centered and conducive to blood and qi flow. Zheng also told us, "The hand is not a hand. Every part of my body is a hand, but hands have nothing to do with it," which I did not understand until relatively recently. Now, I see that all three of these admonitions about hands have the following idea in common:

Consider how hands are expressive of our intention. When we want to pick an item up, a hand reaches out in the direction of the item. When we talk, our hands express our thoughts. In Taijiquan, however, the opposite is true. Hands move because they are on the ends of arms. Arms move because of their connectedness to the trunk of the body, and the trunk moves because of the action of the legs and their connection to the pelvis.

When the wrist is in its centered orientation with subtle extension, a marvelous feeling of unification occurs. That feeling can be extended to the elbow, shoulder, etc., until every part of the body becomes likewise unified. When such connectedness of the whole body occurs, with no intention in the hands, there is no feeling of moving the hands, per se. Instead, the hands move as a result of their connection to the rest of the body and subtle peng.

---

46. *The Essence of T'ai Chi Ch'uan, The Literary Tradition*, Edited by Benjamin Pang-jeng Lo et al., North Atlantic Books, Berkeley, CA, 1985, p. 34.

Unfortunately, many practitioners move their hands with intention, and, when they do Taiji movement, their hands move in the normal, everyday way—not in the Taiji way. When your hands touch an opponent in the everyday way, they telegraph your intention to the opponent, who can easily thwart what you want to do. Instead, when your hands have no intention, not only are you more sensitive to the opponent's intention, but the opponent does not know yours. Thus, it is said:

> *The opponent does not know me, but I know the opponent.*
> —Wang Zong-yue[47]

It should be noted that advanced practitioners sometimes attain special hand shapes for accentuating qi in their hands. These shapes are of much value but should be practiced only after attaining the beauteous wrist, that is, practicing with no intention in the hands.

"ALL MOVEMENT COMES FROM THE WAIST"

This admonition is given because beginners incorrectly tend to move peripherally by twisting the spine, pulling the shoulders, and reaching with the arms, hands, and legs. Instead, all turning movement, which is a major source of propulsion of the limbs, must result from a unified movement of the whole trunk of the body about its axis. However, without the action of the legs, the only movement that the pelvis can make is to tilt forward and backward (about an axis joining the centers of the hip joints). This movement of the pelvis is not what is meant by "All movement comes from the waist." Instead, the turning movement of the pelvis and trunk should come from the bending of one leg and the straightening of the other and from the connection of the thigh bones to the pelvis (kua).

It is important for more-advanced practitioners to concentrate on actually feeling the propulsion of all body parts as originating from the floor, to the centers of the feet, and projecting through the legs, pelvis, spine, arms, and hands in a unified manner. To feel this propulsion, it is necessary to do slow, repetitive, mindful movements involving shifting the weight and turning the body. The key here is having the mind unify all parts of the body with each other.

---

47. Ibid., p. 35.

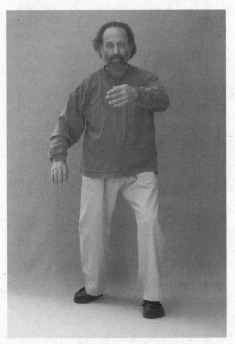

Fig. 5-1. *A photograph of the author in the 70-30 posture "Ward off Left." Note that the head and navel point in the same direction as the forward foot.*

Whereas the main source of powerful movement is through propulsion by the legs, actually, when the body is unified, movement of any part of the body can be assisted by moving any other part. For example, lowering an arm can help turn the body, or bringing a limb closer to the body while it is turning can increase the rate of rotation.

"IN EACH COMPLETED POSTURE, THE NAVEL MUST POINT IN THE DIRECTION OF THE FORWARD FOOT"[48]

Unfortunately, some practitioners do not realize that this admonition only applies to 70-30 postures. In 70-30 postures, the navel *does* point in the direction of the forward foot (see Fig. 5-1). However, in 100% postures where, in Zheng Manqing's style, the weighted foot is at 90 degrees to the direction of the stance, the navel is midway between the directions of the two feet (see Fig. 5-2).[49]

---

48. More precisely, this admonition should say, "In each completed stance, the median plane of the body is parallel to the center line of the forward foot."
49. More precisely, the intersection of the median plane of the body and the horizontal plane bisects the angle between the center lines of the feet.

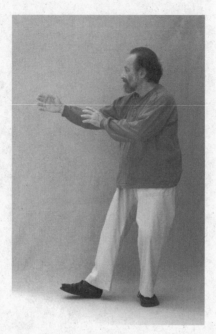

Fig. 5-2. *A photograph of the author in the 100% posture "Raise Hands." Note that the front and rear feet are at 90 degrees (Zheng Manqing's style). The head points in the same direction as the forward foot, but the navel points midway between the direction of the forward foot and that of the rear foot.*

In 100% postures, it is advisable to open the hip joint of the weighted leg but not at the expense of the alignment of that leg. Attempting to open to the point where the navel points in the direction of the forward foot tends to pull the knee of the weighted leg inward, out of its optimal alignment. Optimal alignment occurs in a 100% stance when the knee of the 100%-weighted leg is directly above the center line of that foot (see Fig. 5-3). When the weight is 100% on one leg, trying to open too much pulls the knee inward from that optimal relationship and causes a shear stress on the knee joint; namely, the end of the femur (thigh bone) at the knee joint tends to move inward, and the tibia (shin bone) tends to move outward. This shear leads to stretching of the inner knee ligaments and to consequent pain or even chronic or acute injury. Over time, practicing opening the hip joint of the weighted leg without losing the right alignment will eventually train the hip joint to open more. Based on the indentations of the pelvis and femur, these bones would actually come into contact for an opening of 90°, so it is doubtful that many practitioners can achieve that limit.

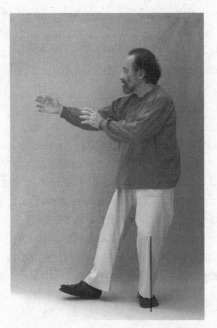

Fig. 5-3. *Optimal alignment occurs in a 100% stance when the knee of the 100%-weighted leg is directly above the center line of that foot, as shown by the plumb line drawn.*

"THE HEAD DOES NOT TURN"

There are two literal and overly simple interpretations of this admonition. One such interpretation is that the head always points in the same direction in space. This interpretation is obviously incorrect because, during Taiji movement, the head faces different directions in space. The other interpretation is that the head does not turn *relative to the body*. The following analysis will reject this latter interpretation.

In 70-30 postures, the nose points in the direction of the navel[50] (see Fig. 5-1). However, in 100% postures, the nose points in the direction of the center line of the forward (empty) foot (see Fig. 5-3). For example, the head doesn't turn relative to the body from "Ward Off Right" through "Single Whip." However, immediately after that, when you make the transition from "Single Whip" to "Raise Hands," the body turns approximately 45° to the right, but the head turns 90° to the right, approximately 45° more than the body (the head turns twice as much as does the body). Therefore, the interpretation that the head does not turn relative to the

---

50. More precisely, the median plane of the head and the median plane of the body are coincident. A *median plane* is a plane that divides the body (or head, etc.) into two symmetric halves. See Fig. 3-1 for definitions of the three bodily planes: median, frontal, and horizontal.

body is incorrect. That the head does not turn is thus another seemingly paradoxical Chinese admonition, which means that there is a deeper meaning to uncover beyond the simple idea that the head is not turning all over the place, independently of the motion of the body.

The admonition becomes clear if you understand that the movement of the head is not the ordinary kind, which uses muscular contraction. Instead, the movement results from muscular extension. That is, the muscles in the neck should be in a slightly extended state (along with every other muscle in the body). This extension protects the neck and head from injury and makes movement of the head much more continuous and able to be metered out. The turning of the head is accomplished by lengthening muscles in the same manner as all other movement that is activated by muscular extension. In fact, the admonition that the head should not turn is similar to the admonition that the hands should not move. In each case, motion occurs not by ordinary means but by muscular extension which is the same as that which causes the head to be as if suspended from above.

"THE HEAD SHOULD ALWAYS STAY AT THE SAME LEVEL"

In both long and short Taiji empty-hand forms, there are movements in which the head obviously does not follow this admonition. Recently, a beginning student under my teacher, Harvey Sober asked, "In doing the form, does the head always stay at the same level?" Sober's answer was, "It does—except when it doesn't." Examples of such atypical movements are "Downward Single Whip," "Downward Punch," and "Needle at Sea Bottom." Some people even purposely change height in additional moves such as in the transition into "Single Whip" just before the final step with the left foot. These anomalous, vertical excursions are done to accentuate the vertical flow of qi in the body, an effect that I experience when doing these movements that way.

Of course, it is necessary for a beginner to first do moves (other than the obvious ones mentioned) at the same level for quite some time in order to know the difference. One must first empty before filling because an empty cup holds the most.

In order to keep the head at the same level when shifting the weight, the knee of the leg onto which the weight is shifting must bend increasingly as weight is shifted onto that leg. Otherwise, the body arcs upward as the weight shifts (see Fig. 5-4).

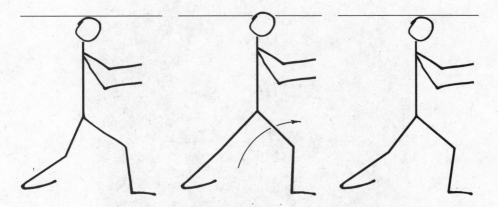

Fig. 5-4. *The person on the left is about to shift forward without moving his feet. The person in the middle has shifted forward without bending his forward knee at all, thus rotating clockwise about the ankle joint of his forward foot, causing his head to rise. The person on the right has shifted by bending her forward knee just the amount that results in her head staying at the same level.*

"The Head is as if Suspended from Above"

An interpretation of this admonition is as follows: The skull is, of course, bone, which rests on the atlas, the uppermost cervical vertebra (see Fig. 5-5). In all, there are seven cervical vertebrae (pronounced *vertibray* or *vertebree*) that lie between the skull and the trunk of the body. The movement of these seven vertebrae control the movement of the head relative to the trunk of the body; the movement of the vertebrae below these top seven does not result in any movement of the head relative to the body. Normally, the head rests on the atlas, which is the top vertebra. The atlas, in turn, rests on the next lower vertebra, and so on. However, in doing Taiji, different conditions exist.

In doing Taiji, the musculature around the cervical vertebrae is in a state of subtle muscular extension. Thus, in Taiji, the skull and each of the cervical vertebrae are subtly extended upward, which gives the head a feeling of being "suspended from above." The state of extension also conduces to completing the greater yang circuit of qi flow and contributes to a general alertness of the spirit.

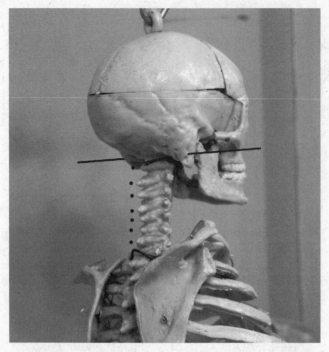

Fig. 5-5. *A photograph of a plastic skeleton showing the seven cervical vertebrae (posterior of each is marked by a dot) that lie between the skull and the trunk of the body. The vertebra just below the black metal clip is the first thoracic vertebra. A horizontal axis is drawn in the frontal plane through the atlas. Note that this line intersects the center of the mastoid processes, which are very easy to feel with your fingers. Here the head is* literally *suspended from above, and the weight of the whole skeleton has straightened out the cervical curve.*

> *An insubstantial energy leads the head [upward].*
> —Anonymous[51]

> *Effortlessly the chin [ji] reaches the headtop.*
> —Wang Tsung-yueh[52]

The following exercise for moving each cervical vertebra independently was taught to me by Elaine Summers:

Exercise: First find the point where the skull rests on the atlas by placing the tip of each forefinger on the mastoid process on each side.

51. Yang, Jwing-Ming, *Tai Chi Secrets of the Ancient Masters*, YMAA Publication Center, Boston, MA, 1999, p. 63.
52. *The Essence of T'ai Chi Ch'uan, The Literary Tradition*, Edited by Benjamin Pang-jeng Lo et al., North Atlantic Books, Berkeley, CA, 1985, p. 40.

Then try to move the head very slightly in each direction about this point, keeping all the cervical vertebrae motionless. Next, move the head and the atlas together about the next lower vertebra. Continue until there are eight separate movements, one for each articulation of the seven cervical vertebrae.

"THE FOOT MUST BE FLAT ON THE GROUND"

A misinterpretation of this admonition is for practitioners to think that every part of the sole of the foot should contact the floor (flatfooted). Consequently, they let their arches cave in, which results in improper alignment of ankles and knees. As I have pointed out in other writings,[53] the integrity of the arch must always be maintained. Collapsing the arch leads to all manner of foot, ankle, and knee problems. Moreover, collapsing the arch makes the body weak for the following reason: When alignment of any part of the body is off, the misaligned parts are vulnerable to injury. When you exert force on an external object or person, the reaction to this force places a stress on your own body, and any misaligned part is placed in danger of being injured. To protect itself, the body will naturally avoid being injured by limiting the amount of force generated. Thus, wrong alignment limits the amount of force you can exert.

What *is* meant by the foot-flat admonition is that in a 70-30 stance, the toe of your forward foot must not lift during a weight shift to the rear and the heel of your rear foot must not lift during a forward weight shift. Many practitioners tend to commit both of these errors. For example, in shifting backward in the transition from "Press" to "Push," it is an error for the toe of the forward foot to come off the floor. Similarly, in shifting forward in the transition from "Press" to "Push," the rear heel should not come off the floor. Once the toe of the forward foot lifts, it is very easy for someone to push you backward. Similarly, once the heel of the rear foot lifts off the ground, it is very easy for someone to pull you forward.

Scientifically stated, at all times, the *relative* distribution of pressure on the sole of your foot must remain constant. Moreover, the center of the distribution of the weight must be centered on the center of the foot

---

53. See Robert Chuckrow, *The Tai Chi Book*, YMAA Publication Center, Boston, MA, 1998, and Robert Chuckrow, *Tai Chi Walking*, YMAA Publication Center, Boston, MA, 2002.

without letting the arch cave in or putting excessive pressure on the front or rear or the inside or outside of the foot. One way to describe this condition is to imagine each foot resting on a board, which, in turn, rests on the pointed end of a vertical stake of wood. In order for each foot to be balanced, the top of each stake would have to be under the center of each foot. Yet, the balance point might be under the arch, which does not make any contact with the board. Nevertheless, the weight distribution on each foot would be centered at the center of that foot.

This criterion of centering the weight on the center of each foot applies to shifting the weight onto or off a foot. The distribution of pressure should remain exactly the same as the weight comes onto or off the foot. That is, as your weight shifts onto a foot, the pressure at each point of the foot will increase, but the manner in which the pressure is distributed should not change. A similar statement applies to shifting your weight off a foot.

The following method of finding the centers of your feet is reproduced from the chapter on alignment of the author's book on Taiji walking:[54]

Optimal balance and alignment of the feet, arches, and ankles are most efficiently experienced by becoming aware of the centers of your feet. I learned the following key relationship from Sam Chin Fan-siong:

The distribution of weight on a foot should be centered on the center of that foot.

This relationship needs to be satisfied for any weight distribution between your two feet. For example, in a 70-30 position (70% on the forward foot and 30% on the rear foot), 70% of your weight is distributed on your forward foot in such a manner that the center of that distribution is located at the center of that foot. A corresponding statement applies to your rear foot.

The following exercise, taught to me by Chin Fan-siong, is useful in locating the centers of your feet:

Exercise: Stand with both feet parallel and comfortably apart, and rock forward and backward. The amplitude of the motion should always be large enough to feel that the center of your weight distribution is alternately forward of and behind what you feel to be the center of your foot. As your sensitivity increases, continually reduce the amplitude of the excursions until you stop at center. If you do this exercise frequently and mindfully, you

---

54. Robert Chuckrow, *Tai Chi Walking*, YMAA Publication Center, Boston, MA, 2002, pp. 23–24.

will eventually know where the center of your foot is in the forward and rear direction.

To find the lateral center of your foot, again stand with the feet parallel. Now alternately bring the knees inward and outward, feeling how the weight shifts from the insides of your feet to the outsides. Again, reduce the excursions until you feel your weight centered on the center lines of the feet.

It is good to alternate the forward and lateral exercises. Do not be surprised if, at first, the centered alignment feels strange. This reaction always accompanies a correction to habitual wrong alignment. Eventually, your body will know and tell you which alignment is valid.

Here is another exercise for improving your awareness of the centers of the feet: Stand with the feet parallel and a comfortable width apart (centers of feet about one-half a pelvis width apart). Try to attain the optimal alignment of the feet just discussed. Bend your knees, and move them in a horizontal circle without moving your feet. Notice that your tibias (shin bones) describe cones with vertices at the ankle joints. Sense the points of the feet below these vertices.

"The Knee Should Not Go Past the Toe"

This admonition is misunderstood in a number of ways. Some people erroneously think that damage to the knee can result from "overextending," and they apply the rule to all postures, even 100% ones. Actually, this admonition applies to 70-30 stances only. In a 70-30 stance, the weight is shared between both legs. If the knee of the forward leg goes past the toe, it becomes fairly easy for an opponent to pull you out of your root. The criterion here has only to do with stability, not with any danger that the knee can be damaged by extending further.

Some say that, in a 70-30 stance, the toe should not go beyond the *root* of the toe. Others say that the shin should not go past vertical in that stance.

For 100% stances, the principle governing how far one should extend the knee has to do primarily with stability. As the knee moves forward, the center of the weight distribution on that foot goes forward of its center, and the weight shifts onto the ball of the foot. As soon as the center of the weight distribution on the foot goes forward of its center, you are overextended and easily pulled forward.

In a 100% stance, depending on the length of the quadriceps, the knee can go way past the toe without damage as long as (1) the muscles and tendons are allowed to strengthen over time and are not stressed beyond their limit and (2) the alignment is correct. Optimal alignment occurs in a 100% stance when the knee of the 100%-weighted leg is directly above the center line of that foot. That relationship requires that the weight distribution on the 100% foot be centered on the center of that foot.

It should be mentioned again that when the weight is 100% on one leg, attempting to open the hip joint too much during turning the body outward pulls the knee of the weighted leg inward from the optimal relationship and causes a shear stress on the knee joint; namely, the end of the femur (thigh bone) at the knee joint tends to move inward, and the tibia (shin bone) tends to move outward. This shear stretches the inner knee ligaments and to consequent pain or even chronic or acute injury. Of course, the more bent the knee of a person with incorrect alignment, the greater the chance of damage in a 100% stance. However, a person need not worry about any harmful effects of lowering the body and extending the knee in a 100% stance as long as alignment is correct and limitations of muscles and tendons are not exceeded. Again, for maximal stability, the center of the distribution of weight on the 100% foot should not go forward of the center of that foot.

If one is only interested in strengthening the legs during form practice, sitting totally into the 100% leg is of use. However, it should be recognized that doing so makes the 100% leg totally yin. In regular practice, establishing the dot of yang in the yin involves a slight extension of the 100% leg.

THE HEAVY/LIGHT PARADOX

Various Taiji writings claim that the arms should be very heavy. Others say that the arms should be very light. The Taijiquan Classics say:

> *A feather cannot be added; nor can a fly alight*
> —Wang Tsung-yueh[55]

This statement is taken to mean that the body should be so delicately balanced and free-moving that a feather will be felt for its weight and that a fly alighting will set the whole body into motion.

---

55. Lee Ying-arng, *Lee's Modified Tai Chi for Health*, Mclisa Enterprises, P.O. Box 1755, Honolulu, Hawaii 96806, 1968, p. 39.

Chen Wei-ming, in his commentary of Yang Cheng-fu's ten important points says, "Someone who has extremely good T'ai Chi Ch'uan *kung fu* has arms like iron wrapped with cotton and the weight is very heavy."[56] The word *heavy* can be interpreted as meaning massive (resistant to changes in motion) or weighty for their gravitational attraction to the earth (what a scale would measure if you stood on it). When the arms are "delicately poised," gravity is neutralized by correct force, so the arms seem light in that an opponent touching them will feel them to be very easily moved but, at the same time, massive because they are connected in a unified manner to every other part of the body. An analogy is a boat floating in the water. It might weigh hundreds of pounds but can be moved with very little force.

"HAN XIONG BA BEI"

含胸拔背

This admonition (*Hán Xīong Bá Bè*) can be translated as "enclose the front, extend the back upward." It is not uncommon for some Taiji practitioners to take this expression so literally that they hunch over, compressing their lungs and internal organs when doing Taiji. Han xiong ba bei really pertains to establishing an appropriate balance of yin and yang. By nature, the front of the body is yin and the back is yang. In Western countries, there is an idea that a man should expand his chest and suck in his gut like a soldier at attention. Expanding the chest throws yin and yang out of balance by making the front of the body, a naturally yin region, yang. The front of the body needs to be supportive and somewhat hollow (both of these qualities are yin), and the back needs to be active and somewhat convex (both of these qualities are yang). Instead of expanding the chest, we need to subtly expand the back, especially the lower back, which is an area that tends to collapse inward (see Fig. 5-6 for a schematic representation of the distinction between the two shapes). The expansion of the back in han xiong ba bei is very slight, and any attempt to shove the body into such an alignment is wrong. Of course, the lower abdomen should be relaxed and allowed to expand naturally.

---

56. *The Essence of T'ai-Chi Ch'uan, The Literary Tradition,* Edited by Benjamin Pang-jeng Lo, North Atlantic Books, Berkeley, CA, 1985, p. 87.

Even though the front of the body is yin, there is a dot of yang, which is a subtle active extension of the front of the body. This frontal support allows the back to relax any contractive action, which can be though of as the dot of yin in the yang in the back.

When you push an object or a person, by Newton's third law (action and reaction), the reaction to the force you exert is an equal force back on you. This reaction force tends to bend your body backward to the shape shown on the right side of figure 5-6. An untrained person will avoid bending backward by contracting the muscles in the front of his body. Such a use of contractive force inhibits natural breathing, rigidifies the body, can only be held for a short time without tiring, compromises rooting, and is difficult to modify with changing conditions. Maintaining the outward shape of han xiong ba bei with incorrect muscular action (frontal contraction) has similar disadvantages. However, maintaining han

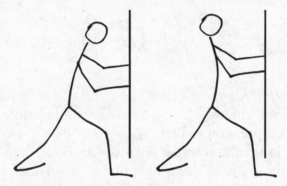

Fig. 5-6. *The person on the left is pushing an object correctly (han xiong ba bei). The person on the right has his back concave and front convex, contrary to han xiong ba bei. It is obvious which way of pushing is more effective.*

xiong ba bei by extending the muscles in the back of the body and emptying the front of contractive force allows natural breathing, makes the body resilient and unified, can be sustained for a relatively long time, augments rooting, and is easy to change with changing conditions.

Consider the forces on a person pushing on an object (Fig. 5-7). Let us first assume that the person's body is upright. The reaction to the force F_{OP} on the object by the person is a force F_{PO} on the person by the object (see "Newton's Third Law" in Ch. 4).[57] The two frictional forces F_{Pf1} and

---

57. Note that the first subscript refers to the entity on which the force is exerted, and the second subscript refers to the entity exerting the force.

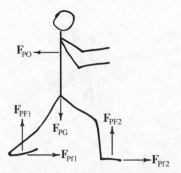

Fig. 5-7. *The forces on a person pushing an object.* $\mathbf{F}_{PO}$ *is the force on the person by the object,* $\mathbf{F}_{PG}$ *is the force on the person by gravity,* $\mathbf{F}_{Pf1}$ *and* $\mathbf{F}_{Pf2}$ *on the person by the floor on the person's rear foot and front, respectively, and* $\mathbf{F}_{PF1}$ *and* $\mathbf{F}_{PF2}$ *are the upward forces on the person by the floor.*

$\mathbf{F}_{Pf2}$ on the person by the floor on the person's rear foot and front, respectively, balance $\mathbf{F}_{PO}$ and prevent the person from sliding backward. In addition, $\mathbf{F}_{PO}$ tends to bend the person's body backward and rotate it backward about the rear foot. The untrained person will prevent bending backward by maintaining contractive tension in the front of his body. As $\mathbf{F}_{PO}$ builds up, $\mathbf{F}_{PF2}$ automatically reduces, and backward rotation is prevented to the degree that the force of gravity on the person's body counteracts the backward-rotational-effect of $\mathbf{F}_{PO}$. Thus, stability is limited by the person's contractive strength and his weight.

But what if the rotational effect of the force on the person by the object is greater than that of gravity? Then, even if the person's body does not bend, it will rotate backward as a rigid system. Or, what if the external force is suddenly removed? Then the person will lose stability and fall forward because the contracted muscles will not immediately release their pull.

Now consider what happens if the person is not necessarily heavy and not particularly strong in a conventional sense but assumes a state of han xiong ba bei. The additional internal forces, $\mathbf{F}_u$ and $\mathbf{F}_d$ resulting from han xiong ba bei act like the expansion of steam in the cylinders of a locomotive (see Fig. 5-8). These forces stabilize the person and prevent bending backward. Next, the person in a state of han xiong ba bei, by using correct force, will also be more able to maintain stability should $\mathbf{F}_{PO}$ suddenly disappear. Finally, by the person pushing the object slightly upward, the object's force $\mathbf{F}_{PO}$ on the person now is downward, which provides the following benefits: (1) The horizontal component of $\mathbf{F}_{PO}$ is now less than

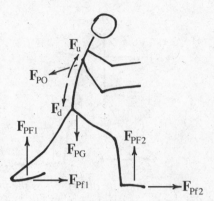

Fig. 5-8. *The additional upward and downward internal forces* F_u *and* F_d, *respectively, on a person in han xiong ba bei.*

before, which produces less of a backward-rotational effect on the person. (2) Because the horizontal component of F_{PO} is now less than before, the frictional forces F_{Pf1} and F_{Pf2} will now need to be less. (3) Now there is a downward vertical component of F_{PO}, which increases F_{PF1}, allowing the frictional force F_{Pf1} to be larger than before[58] (even though it now needs to be less).

   If the person in han xiong ba be is pushing a partner instead of an inanimate object, the person's force on the partner will be slightly upward, causing the partner to experience the reverse of two of the beneficial effects just enumerated. Namely, the person's force on the partner will lift him out of his root and produce *more* of a backward-rotational effect on him (see Fig. 5-9). These effects weaken the partner and make it easier to uproot him.

Exercises: A good way to practice han xiong ba bei is to exert a gentle force against a wall in the "Push" posture, paying particular attention to the modes of muscular action in the front and back of the body. As your han xiong ba bei increases in strength, you can exert increased force on the wall. Later, you can practice using "Ward Off." Once you have achieved correct han xiong ba bei, to should be subtly incorporated into all movements during regular practice of the Taiji form and push-hands.

---

58. When two objects are in contact, the maximum frictional force between them is proportional to the force with which the surfaces are pressed together. In this case, the surfaces are the floor and the person's foot.

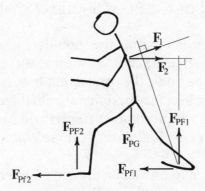

Fig. 5-9. *Comparison of the leverage effects of differently directed forces* $\mathbf{F}_1$ *and* $\mathbf{F}_2$. *It can be seen that the perpendicular distance from the center of the rear foot to the line of* $\mathbf{F}_1$ *is greater than that to* $\mathbf{F}_2$. *Thus,* $\mathbf{F}_1$ *has more leverage about the rear foot than* $\mathbf{F}_2$.

"THE SPINE IS HELD STRAIGHT, AND THE BODY SHOULD NOT LEAN"

Some interpret this admonition to mean that the axis of the body is always vertical, and others that the axis of the body may tilt forward at a substantial angle as long as the spine does not bend from its optimal alignment. Anyone who has practiced the martial applications of the Taiji movements knows that the body needs to lean into the direction of the application of force on an opponent. Were the body perfectly upright at the instant of a strike, the reaction to the force exerted would bend and rotate the body backwards, which would make the body weak.

The question is whether there should be any leaning in doing movements of the form, where the application of force is only implied. Some practitioners believe that one purpose of practicing the form is to cultivate a body mechanic that would apply in a real situation, so they lean. Others believe that, when playing with the air, there is no need to attain a state that is required only for the exertion of a large force and that the body should only lean in proportional to a physical need to do so, so they strive to stay upright.

One of the most important benefits in doing the form is to learn to relax contractive strength. Relaxing when leaning is very difficult, especially for a beginner. But leaning while doing the form can be of value once you have sufficiently developed correct strength (but not before).

"The Trunk of the Body Should not Twist"

The word *twist* means that in turning, the shoulders turn a different amount (usually more) than the pelvis. As soon as there is any active twisting of the trunk of the body, the connection between top and bottom is lost, and the movement becomes peripheral and, therefore, weak. Most beginners and even some advanced practitioners will incorrectly twist their bodies in such moves as "Roll Back," "Single Whip," and "Step Back to Repulse the Monkey."

However, once you learn to move in a unified manner, with all parts rotating the same amount, you will find that a relaxed body *does* twist— but passively, not actively. The reason is that once there is a certain amount of rotational velocity of the body, when the pelvis comes to a stop, the top of the body will keep rotating slightly because of its rotational inertia. By the same token, the twisted body has a spring-like potential energy (called *torsional potential energy*). When unleashed at the instant desired, the torsional potential energy causes the body to begin rotation in the opposite direction.

6

Stretching

The concepts presented in this chapter were taught to me primarily by Elaine Summers.

BENEFITS OF STRETCHING

Proper stretching activates muscles, tendons, bones, organs, glands, blood vessels, acupuncture meridians, nerves, and flow of lymph. The beneficial stresses placed on bones while stretching encourage them to absorb nutrients that increase their density and strength. While you are stretching, your mind tends to enter a mode in which it is experiencing directly rather than through words and other's ideas, prejudices, etc. This mode is a precursor for meditation.

One important dividend of stretching regularly is developing a sense of your body's range of flexibility and state of well-being. Any improvement or deterioration is promptly noticed and can then be traced to its cause in the immediate past. That cause can be repeated if its result is beneficial or avoided if its result is harmful. Without such a bodily sense, injurious actions are not connected with their effects and often continue unabated.

Finally, stretching by using muscular extension is a way of developing the use of correct force in doing Taiji movement and push-hands.

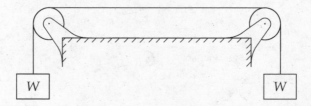

Fig. 6-1. *When a wire is subjected to a force on each end (here caused by the hanging weights, each of weight W), it causes an amount of tension in the wire equal to W. If, for example, each weight is 10 pounds, then the tension in the wire is 10 pounds (not 20 pounds!).*

WAYS OF STRETCHING

Passive Stretching

To stretch an inanimate object means lengthening it by applying a force on each end, away from center (see Fig. 6-1 for an analogous physical system). The type of stress thus caused is called *tensile stress* or *tension*.

(1) Gravity and leverage can cause muscles to lengthen (e.g., standing with feet parallel and slightly apart, bending forward, lowering the upper body, and allowing it to hang). Gravity is natural and very predictable. These features make it easy for you to relax and give in to gravity's effects. Thus, stretching by allowing gravity and leverage to lengthen muscles can be of value if done cautiously.

(2) Passive stretching can occur when momentum or centrifugal effects lengthen muscles. These quantities come into play in a very gentle manner in doing the Taiji form.

(3) Massage and chiropractic manipulation can be thought of as involving passive stretching.

(4) Another way to stretch is to allow another person to apply force to lengthen your muscles and tendons. Sometimes such stretching is done using another person's body weight. Allowing another person's idea of what your body is capable of plus that person's unpredictable application of strength can cause serious injury and is not recommended.

Active Stretching

When we deal with a human body whose muscles can actively shorten or lengthen, *stretching* can now mean any one of the following:

(1) One set of muscles contracts, causing tension in that set of muscles and associated tendons. The opposing set of muscles are passively caused to become longer (stretched) whether they "want to" or not. Lengthening muscles mercilessly by contracting the opposing set of muscles is a bad practice because it programs a way of moving that can cause injury during a sudden movement. Pitting one set of muscles against another is antithetical to all principles of doing things naturally at a natural rate.

(2) The muscles that get longer do so by their own extension rather than by being forced to do so by other muscles and possibly leverage. Stretching muscles by extending them not only will tone and lengthen them but will also help you to cultivate "correct force."

(3) Using momentum in a spirited manner (e.g., standing with feet parallel, letting the upper body hang, and lifting and bouncing) is permissible only if the muscles and tendons involved are in a high degree of tone and strength.

USING MUSCULAR EXTENSION FOR STRETCHING

The key to proper stretching is to actively lengthen the side getting longer rather than contracting the opposite side. For example, consider the action of tilting your head to the left so that your left ear moves toward your left shoulder. This action should result from lengthening the muscles on the *right* side of your neck rather than contracting the muscles on the left side (see Fig. 6-2).

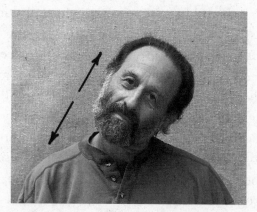

Fig. 6-2. *Stretching by lengthening the muscles (in the direction of the arrows) on the side that is getting longer.*

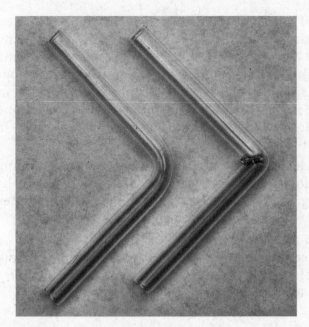

Fig. 6-3. *Two lengths of glass tubing, each of which was bent 90° in a different manner. The tubing on the left was correctly bent by applying heat primarily on the outside of the bend, thus causing that part to lengthen. The tubing on the right was incorrectly bent by applying heat primarily on the inside of the bend, thus causing that part to constrict.*

An analogy is the way a glass blower bends glass tubing. If a flame is applied to one side of the tubing and the glass is bent away from that side, the glass stretches. By contrast, if the glass is bent toward the heated side, the glass collapses on the inside of the bend. Figure 6-3 shows two lengths of glass tubing that I bent 90° to illustrate the principle involved. In addition to bending the tubing away from the heated side, I applied controlled air pressure to the inside of the tubing at one end, temporarily keeping the other end sealed. This pressure helped to keep the outside of the curve expanded. Of course, the glass tubing cannot move on its own, whereas your body can. Nevertheless, the example still illustrates the principle of expanding and lengthening the side turned away from.

We are very much in the habit of bossing our bodies around. Of course, our bodies need to be subservient to our wishes, otherwise we would get little done. But when mindful movement is done in the name of health, and that movement programs into our daily actions a way of using our bodies, the way that movement is done is crucial. If we boss our bodies around in the name of exercise, we might feel virtuous, but all we are doing is compounding the harm that is done by all the other movement of that sort during the day.

The key is to allow our bodies to move the way they naturally will if allowed. An analogy is taking a dog that lives in an apartment all day to a grassy area and removing its leash, allowing it to run joyfully. When we unleash our own natural movement, it will always involve muscular extension. Doing so is not only beneficial, but capturing the feeling of such movement teaches us how to introduce it into the Taiji movements.

When we yawn and do movement associated with yawning, we are using muscular extension. Therefore, a good way of doing stretching is to start with a yawn and let the associated feeling pervade the body as movement is done.

STRETCHING USING THE FLOOR

Elaine Summers told me that, early on in her studies, she realized that doing movement while lying on the floor had important advantages. One advantage is that there is no necessity to deal with balance and the effects of gravity. Another advantage is that you are more able to let go of your preconceptions of how you "hold" and move your body. In just about every class that I had with her, most of the time was spent with me lying on the floor and moving very slowly under her watchful eyes. Every so often Summers would say such things as, "Good!" or, "You are using your ribs a lot. Try moving by using the muscles around your spine."

HOW TO RISE TO STANDING AFTER STRETCHING ON THE FLOOR

After lying on the floor for a period of time, even if you are not doing any movement but especially if you are, your muscles have naturally gone beyond their accustomed length. At that time, it is crucial not to place any stress on them when arising. To do so can damage them. Also, it is like punishing your body for letting itself be coaxed into relaxing and moving naturally. Next time, your body will be less agreeable to releasing its habitual tensions. Also, by rising from the floor haphazardly, your muscles will jump back to their old tensions and patterns of usage. Much of the benefit from stretching will have been undermined because you will not experience your muscles in their longer, more-relaxed state while standing.

The following way of rising from the floor after stretching is advised: Slowly roll onto one side, and use your arms instead of the muscles around the spine to come up to sitting on your heels (or other way of sitting) for a short time. Then, slowly come up to standing, recreating the relaxed, heavy feeling that you have when rising from a hot bath.

Rule: Whenever muscles have spent time in an unaccustomed range of their motion, no stress should be placed on them until they have had sufficient time to recover their normal tone.

7

Push-Hands

Today's world is characterized by an ever-increasing tendency toward reckless, impulsive, and extreme behavior. Doing push-hands correctly has the potential for reducing this tendency in ourselves. It also trains us to be less likely to attract others' negativity and to deflect it should it be directed toward us. Note that the fundamentals of push-hands are covered in a separate book.[59]

WINNING

Winning and losing are meaningful in terms of combat or a competition. Push-hands practice is neither winning nor losing. In discussing two-person practice, Ninjutsu teacher, Kevin Harrington, said, "If your partner loses, you lose too." The push-hands players have come together for one purpose, namely to learn. As soon as any thought of winning occurs, the practice has become clouded. At that point, principles of Taiji are sacrificed, and one resorts to brute strength, impulsiveness, learned techniques, and preconceived action. Non-action, being in the moment, balancing yin and yang, and correct strength then go out the window. Doing push-hands to win is to forsake true development for an illusion of having made progress. It is feeding the ego for a short-lived, false feeling of accomplishment but losing an opportunity to learn something that will persist and grow.

---

59. See Robert Chuckrow, *The Tai Chi Book*, YMAA Publication Center, Boston, MA, 1998 and Robert Chuckrow, *Tai Chi Walking*, YMAA Publication Center, Boston, MA, 2002, Ch. 11.

OVERCOMING ONE-THOUSAND
POUNDS USING FOUR OUNCES

The concept that four ounces is all that is needed to deflect a force of 1,000 pounds is well-known to Taiji push-hands practitioners. The following quote is noteworthy: "A student asked about the meaning of 4 oz. Professor [Zheng] replied: 'Indeed, 4 oz. cannot deflect one thousand pounds. But there is a key word—*leading*. (Chinese word: Chan-1) If a cow weighs one thousand pounds and a rope on the cow's nose weighs 4 oz., a boy can walk the cow with the rope. But if the rope is on [the] cow's leg, do you think the cow will go with the boy? In practicing push-hands, it is for us to find out where is the cow's leg and where is the nose.'"[60]

Another aspect of "overcoming one-thousand pounds using four ounces," according to Zheng, is that there is a limit to the effectiveness of four ounces for a very strong attack. For such an attack, the defense may have to involve "receiving energy."[61] Receiving energy means allowing the attacker's force to be applied, causing your legs to bend and store energy beyond that corresponding to your body weight. Then that energy can be returned to the attacker. Receiving energy requires very strong legs and split-second timing.

What some practitioners do not know is that four ounces applies only to the deflection—not to the push. Unfortunately, some practitioners think that if they push with more than four ounces, they are breaking a fundamental principle. Not true! Zheng Manqing, who was famous for his "soft" pushing-hands skills, said of the four ounces of deflection and the force of the push, "Only four ounces of leading force is needed. The power of the push is up to me."[62] That is, the neutralization should involve only four ounces, but the push can involve any amount of force. Of course, all force exerted in Taiji must be jin and not li (this distinction is explained in Chapter 1)! Moreover, the minimum force should always be used.

---

60. From *http://www.wuweitaichi.com/articles/Professor_Cheng_Words.htm*, *The Tao of Taijiquan*, by Sheng-lun Culture & Publishing Co., Taipei, Taiwan, ISBN 957-9273-02-2, 1985, Translated by David Chen, 1999, p. 402.

61. See Cheng Man-ch'ing, *T'ai Chi Ch'uan: A Simplified Method of Calisthenics for Health & Self Defense*, North Atlantic Books, Berkeley, CA, 1981, p.p. 124–125.

62. Cheng Man-ch'ing, *Cheng Tzu's Thirteen Treatises on T'ai Chi Ch'uan*, North Atlantic Books, Berkeley, CA, 1985, P. 94.

USE OF MINIMUM FORCE

In push-hands practice, it is important to break your partner's root before executing a push and then time your push to use the minimum force. That way you will refine your skill in pushing.

A comparison can be made between using extra strength in push-hands and in steering a car. Those who drive a car without power steering, of necessity, drive in a manner that requires the minimum amount of muscle power. For example, they avoid turning the steering wheel when the car is stationary, which takes a lot of strength but would be very easy with power steering. Then, when driving a car with power steering, they carry over that way of driving with minimum assistance of the power-steering unit. By contrast, those with no experience in driving a car without power steering have little or no feeling of just how much they are relying on its power, which they squander. The result is unnecessary strain on the entire steering mechanism and the necessity for frequent repairs. Analogously, if you are very strong and habituated to using that strength, you will tend to use that strength unnecessarily at the expense of gaining sensitivity. However, even though you may be strong, if you limit the use of your strength to the minimum required, your sensitivity and refinement will continually increase. This analysis accounts for those who have little strength attaining a higher skill level in push-hands than those who have strength to spare and use that strength indiscriminately.

DEVELOPING CORRECT STRENGTH

As one who has logged many hours developing strength during push-hands practice, I am familiar with and acknowledge the value of following this route. In this mode of practice, each partner tries to dislodge the other's root by using "relaxed" force. Both partners sink their weight into their feet and try to become immovable when the other starts to push using correct force. Some have disparagingly characterized this modality of practice as "Mongolian wrestling."

Some players do a lot of movement during this type of practice, but others barely move at all. The benefit of practicing strength is the development of a strong root and high degree of implied strength in a situation where only light force is used. A pitfall, however, is that, in the process, sensitivity may be forsaken, and using excessive strength can become habitual. The solution is to practice a variety of modalities from softness and evasiveness to development of correct strength. It is very important to balance these modalities and modify them appropriately when practicing with partners who prefer practicing a given modality.

YIN AND YANG IN PUSH-HANDS

When two people do push-hands, each person's movement undergoes a yin/yang alternation, which reciprocates with that of the other. The person pushing is yang, which is active, expansive, and advancing forward. The person being pushed is yin, which is passive, receptive, and moving backward.

Many people who do push-hands maintain a yang aspect throughout. That is, instead of allowing themselves to be pushed back (yin), they retreat actively, which is yang. When my partner retreats actively, I am often able to execute a nice push because he has drawn me into his space and is committed to a backward motion.

Instead of pulling back (yang), allow your partner to push you back (yin). The use of peng to prevent the outstretched arm from collapsing (dot of yang in the yin), and the loosening of the thigh, knee, and ankle joints, allow you to move backward without your partner needing to apply much force.

As you move back, your yin gradually changes to yang by turning in such a manner that your partner's push is neutralized. At that point, your partner becomes yin and you become yang. The dot of yin in the yang when you push is the readiness to let up when resistance (yang) is felt, thereby supporting your partner and controlling his balance.

RECEIVING AND PROCESSING OF SENSE DATA

In most situations, we utilize the sense data that comes into our eyes to form a mental picture of reality. The processing of such visual sense data tends to be slow because it uses the part of the brain that deals with abstract information such as language. If you rely mainly on your vision in a push-hands or self-defense situation, by the time visual sense data is received and processed and the resulting nerve impulses are sent to the corresponding muscles for initiating a physical response, the situation to which you are responding will have already changed. In short, if you rely mainly on your vision, you will be in the past.

In order to respond to situations spontaneously and appropriately, you must feel with the entire body—not just the eyes but the hands, the skin, and even an as-yet-unnamed sixth sense, which involves a direct awareness of your partner's intention. Such *direct* processing is almost instantaneous and allows you to be in the moment.

PUSH-HANDS ERRORS

Many people with whom I have done push-hands make a number of errors. Some of their errors enable me to uproot them, whereas other of their errors enable them to uproot me. The object of push-hands is not winning but inculcating correct principles. Here are the errors that seem prevalent:

(1) Your partner contrives you to move a certain way so that he can use a preconceived attack such as hooking his arm under your upper arm and pulling you off balance.

(2) Your partner pushes you, using brute strength, before you have lost your balance.

(3) Your partner uses contractive strength rather than muscular extension.

(4) Your partner confuses yin and yang—pulling back rather than moving back because of your push.

(5) Your partner is not in a state of song, so getting him or her off balance is not sufficiently challenging.

(6) Your partner pushes into your strength.

(7) Your partner allows his arm to collapse without any motion of his body as you push him ("lost motion").

(8) Your partner accelerates to get an advantage that would be impossible were everything done at normal speed. Accelerating (speeding up relative to the motion of your partner) is, in effect, being in the future and results from intention to have a preconceived response. It should be kept in mind that in push-hands practice, movement is slowed-down as compared to a fighting situation, where attacks can be lightening fast. Speeding up is unrealistic because, in a fighting situation, there is a limit to the speed that can be attained. Instead, in a fighting situation, the opponent's movements are to be matched by yours. The best way to practice matching your movement to an opponent is to practice

doing so with a partner. Accelerating is usually a result of wanting to win but sacrifices an opportunity for learning.

(9) Your partner breaks the connection between you and him in order to get an advantage.

(10) Your partner uses the same preconceived technique each time independently of what you do.

(11) Your partner uses his/her eyes rather than hands to receive sense data.

DEALING WITH OTHERS' ERRORS

Ideally, push-hands practice should involve some mutual discussion so that both partners learn from each other and from the interaction. When my partner does not want to engage in any verbal exchange, I, nevertheless, feel that it is valuable to continue to deal with what I believe to be his or her errors. However, I terminate practice if I am concerned that one of us will become injured or if practice is a waste of time and results in generating unpleasant feelings.

The following quote is noteworthy: "A student complained about other students pushed [*sic*] him too hard. Professor [Zheng] said: 'Taijiquan is about self-evaluation. Never blame others for being too strong, or too rough, or not following the principles; if you could sense and follow their actions, how could you feel the pushes were too hard?' "[63]

MAINTAINING THE CONNECTION BETWEEN YOU AND YOUR PARTNER

Even before two people touch hands, a mental connection has been made, and when their hands actually touch, a physical element is added to that connection. That connection, however, will be broken if a partner is not in the present moment but in the past or future. It is said that the Yang family practiced two-person movement with each partner holding opposite ends of a thread. One partner would try to break the thread by doing any manner of movement. The other partner would strive to maintain a legendary four-ounce tension in the thread at all times. Then the partners would swap roles.

---

63. From *http://www.wuweitaichi.com/articles/Professor_Cheng_Words.htm*, *The Tao of Taijiquan*, by Sheng-lun Culture & Publishing Co., Taipei, Taiwan, ISBN 957-9273-02-2, 1985, Translated by David Chen, 1999, p. 310.

Story.[64] One day, Yang Cheng-fu received a visit from a martial-arts teacher and several of his disciples. Yang immediately knew that the teacher was highly skilled and intended to challenge him. Realizing that he or the challenger could be severely injured, Yang acted quickly to avert any violence. He held up a length of light cotton thread and asked the visitor to hold the other end, challenging him to try to break the thread with any amount of force. Such a method of testing skill had, until then, been only used as a secret training tool.

At first, the visitor had one of his disciples try, but the disciple had no success. Next the teacher tried. No matter what the teacher did or how fast he moved, Yang allowed no slack in the thread or visible change in its tension. Finally, the teacher, out of breath and drenched in sweat, gave in to Yang, who had remained calm throughout. After that, the two men became friends, and no one was injured.

Capturing Your Partner's Balance

I experienced this high level of skill a few times from Professor Zheng. I remember when I was a beginning student in push-hands, Professor Zheng asked me to touch his shoulder. Even though I did so very gently, the next thing I knew was that I was flying through the air. I had no idea of how it happened—it was as though a puff of air had lifted me. In retrospect, decades later, I realized that he was able to receive my energy even though I had exerted such a small force on him. I can only imagine the result had I committed to a large force!

Here is my present (and obviously limited) understanding of how Zheng was able to accomplish such skillful pushes. As soon as you touched Zheng, he would move back very slightly, neutralizing your force and causing you to momentarily lose your balance. Before you could regain your balance on your own, Zheng would provide your balance by supporting you. Everything occurred with such subtlety, perfect timing, and control of force that you would not realize that Zheng now controlled your balance. He then could let up at any time, causing you to fall toward him. As you exerted contractive force on him to regain your balance, he would sense a wave of tension in your body, and that is when he would push you. You would become airborne but have little feeling of having even been touched.

---

64. See *http://www.geocities.com/meiyingsheng/story.html*, in which this amazing story, by Dr. Mei Ying-sheng, is translated in rich detail by Ted W. Knecht.

USING LEVERAGE

Every active movement done by a human body requires leverage. It is important to understand leverage when exerting force on another person, albeit relatively small in push-hands. Because the human body is three-dimensional, the fulcrum is really a fixed axis about which the body rotates rather than a point.

If the fulcrum is in the wrong place, the action will be ineffectual. Therefore, it is essential to develop an awareness of the placement of the fulcrum used for each movement in push-hands. For example, when your partner exerts force on a part of your body, and the fulcrum (fixed axis) is close to that part, your partner will need to exert a large force to move the point of contact, and that point will only move a small amount. Your exertion of force on your partner by the other side of your body will undergo large movement. Similarly, when your partner exerts force on a part of your body, and the fulcrum (fixed axis) is far from that part, your partner will need to exert a small force to move the point of contact, and that point will have a large motion. Your exertion of force on your partner by the other side of your body will undergo small movement with large force. The choice is yours.

SHAPE (ROUNDNESS)

One day, Zheng had a student use his two arms as calipers to measure the distance of Zheng's waist from front to back. Then Zheng rotated 90° in each direction without the student moving his hands. It was seen that Zheng's midsection was essentially circular. I wondered about the reason for this demonstration and now think that he was showing how a Taiji practitioner's body should feel to an opponent; namely, any force exerted except exactly on dead center causes the body to turn, deflecting the applied force. My guess is that Zheng was not showing anything about his physical shape but that if someone tried to exert force on him, it was *as though* he were perfectly round. Any turning motion would deflect the incoming force. To get the feeling of this type of deflection, use the tips of your fingers to try pushing a 70-pound heavy bag used for practicing strikes and kicks. If you push it anywhere other than dead center, the bag will turn, and your fingers will slip off.

8

Self-Defense Applications of Some Taiji Movements

When I started studying Taiji, there was little mention of it as a martial art, and the martial aspect, did not enter my awareness as I practiced. I even rationalized that the movement, "Punch," was so named only because it *resembled* a fighting move. It was inconceivable to me that such slow, relaxed movement could ever have any self-defense value.

Later, when I was shown some of the "fighting" applications, I began to face a dilemma: It was hard for me to reconcile that something so peaceful and uplifting was potentially violent. As time passed, I became intrigued by the martial aspect but, nevertheless, wondered how to reconcile the seeming disparity between spirituality, health, and healing, on one hand, and martial arts, on the other hand. Certainly, skill in hand-to-hand combat is not often necessary in today's world. The statistics bear out that heart disease, cancer, automobile accidents, and side-effects of pharmaceuticals are far more likely to cause death or injury than being attacked by another person or harmed by a knife or firearm.

But I now understand that health, martial arts, and self-development are not separate—they are interconnected and augment each other. Part of this understanding has emerged from seeing the gentleness and spiritual development yet martial adeptness of some of my teachers. Also, I observed that the teachers I have had with the most awesome martial ability were able to heal broken bones in several weeks and manifest other impressive knowledge of healing.

It was not simply that I just got used to health, martial arts, and self-development spoken about and taught as a whole. It really is that my experience over the decades convinces me that neglecting any one of these three aspects limits progress in the others. In short, I have had teachers who have emphasized self-defense much more than I, but I know that, without my exposure to self-defense, I would not have achieved the progress I have made in the other areas of Taiji.

When reading this chapter, it is important to keep in mind that any practice of an application is to learn natural movement and illustrate certain possibilities in a self-protection situation. In Taiji, there are no techniques, and, therefore, there can be myriad applications for a given movement of the Taiji form. Consequently, the applications next shown are by no means definitive.

Please note the use of peng throughout. Also, the defenses do not involve grabbing the attacker's wrist. Instead, subtle contact is made with the palm, wrist, forearm, upper arm, and, in one case, the thumb (Fig. 8-20). In practicing an application, whenever a need to "muscle" your partner arises, it is necessary to stop and find a way to achieve the result effortlessly. Mutual cooperation and dialogue is of value in that regard.

"WARD OFF LEFT"

B stands with feet naturally apart in a neutral 50-50 stance. Attacker *A* steps forward with his right foot and punches *B* with his right hand. Just before the punch hits *B*, he shifts his weight onto his left foot and turns to the right, thereby avoiding getting hit. At the same time *B* interposes his right wrist between himself and *A*'s punching hand. *B*'s wrist rotates counterclockwise, allowing the punching arm to roll and continue its forward movement (Fig. 8-1). Next, *B* shifts onto his right foot and steps forward, using the back of his left wrist to strike *A*'s ribs under his punching arm (Fig. 8-2).

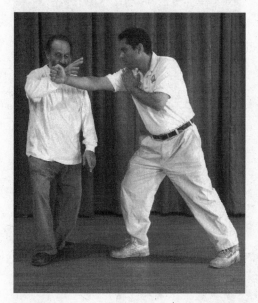 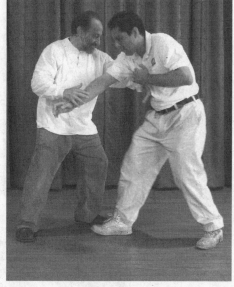

Fig. 8-1   Fig. 8-2

"Roll Back and Press"

B and *A* face each other in harmonious 70-30 stances, both with, say, right feet forward. *A* attacks *B*'s chest with both hands. *B* shifts back, and his arms rise so that his left forearm is between *A*'s arms, and his right forearm is outside *B*'s left forearm (Fig. 8-3). *B* then turns to the left, causing *A* to lose balance (Fig. 8-4). Then *A* shifts forward and turns to the right into "Press" posture (Fig. 8-5).

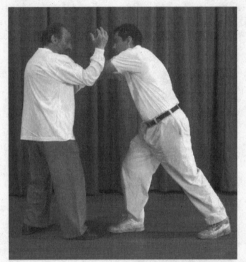

Fig. 8-3

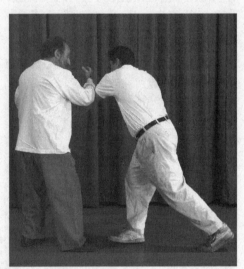

Fig. 8-4

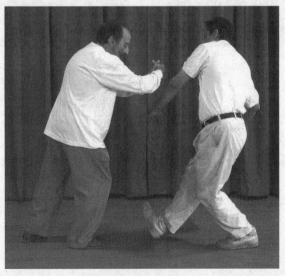

Fig. 8-5

"WITHDRAW AND PUSH"

B stands with feet naturally apart in a neutral 50-50 stance. Attacker *A* steps forward with his right foot and tries to grab *B*'s shirt with both hands (Fig. 8-6). As *A* moves toward *B*, *B* steps back with his left foot. At the same time, *B*'s arms rise under those of *A*. As *B* shifts backward, his arms rotate to palms outward, causing *A* to roll toward *B* on *B*'s arms like packages roll into a supermarket off a truck (Fig. 8-7). Then *B* strikes *A*'s chest with both palms or simply pushes *A* backward (Fig. 8-8).

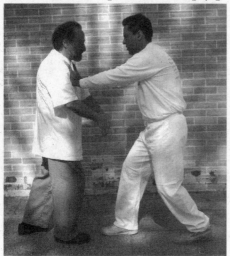

Fig. 8-6

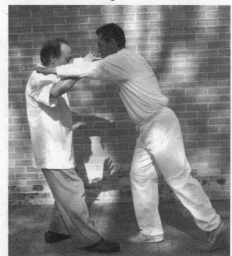

Fig. 8-7

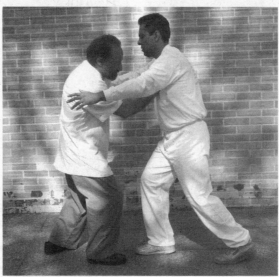

Fig. 8-8

"RAISE HANDS"

B stands with feet naturally apart in a neutral 50-50 stance. Attacker *A* steps forward with his right foot and reaches for *B*'s throat with his right hand. *B* steps back with his left foot, turning to the left. At the same time, *B*'s left wrist comes up outside *A*'s right wrist and rolls *A*'s wrist downward and outward. At the same time *B*'s right wrist rises under *A*'s elbow, locking it (Fig. 8-9). *A* can then turn to the right, attacking *B*'s right elbow, breaking his balance (Fig. 8-10), and then striking *B*'s head with his left hand (Fig. 8-11)

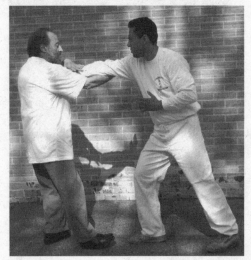

Fig. 8-9

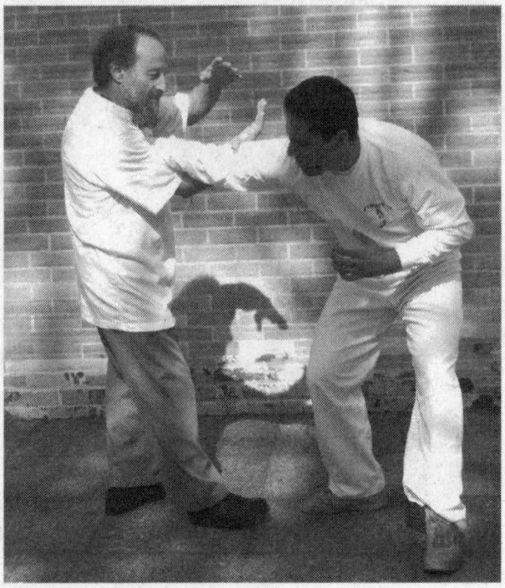

Fig. 8-10

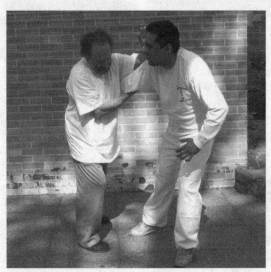

Fig. 8-11

"Strike with Shoulder"

B stands with feet naturally apart in a neutral 50-50 stance. Attacker A steps forward with his right foot and tries to grab B's shirt with both hands. As A moves toward B, B steps back with his right foot, turning to the right. At the same time, B's right arm dives down over the inside of A's left arm (Fig. 8-12), and B's left arm rises on the inside of A's right arm. Then B steps forward with his right foot and strikes A's sternum with his right shoulder (Fig. 8-13).

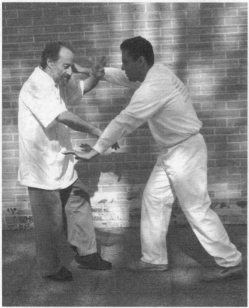

Fig. 8-12

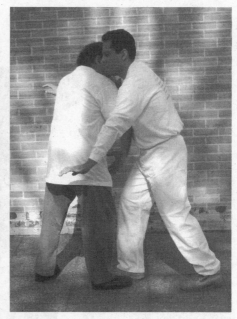

Fig. 8-13

"WHITE CRANE"

B stands with feet naturally apart in a neutral 50-50 stance. Attacker *A* steps forward with his right foot and tries to grab *B*'s shirt with both hands. As *A* moves toward *B*, *B* steps back with his right foot, turning to the right. At the same time, *B*'s left arm dives down over the inside of *A*'s right arm and rotates *A*'s left arm downward and outward, and *B*'s right arm rises on the inside of *A*'s left arm and rotates *A*'s left arm upward and outward. Then *B* kicks *A* with his left foot (Fig. 8-14). Then *B* strikes *A*'s head with his right hand (Fig. 8-15). The beginning of this application is almost the mirror image of "Strike with Shoulder."

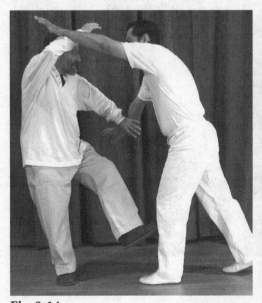
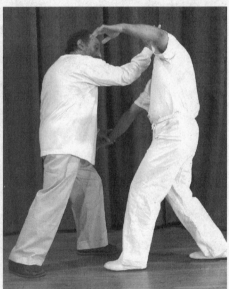

Fig. 8-14   **Fig. 8-15**

"Brush Knee"

B stands with feet naturally apart in a neutral 50-50 stance. Attacker A steps forward and punches B with his right hand. As A moves toward B, B steps back with his right foot, turns to the right, and deflects A's attack with his left forearm (Fig. 8-16). B steps forward with his left foot, and circles A's punching arm downward and pinning A's right hand to his right knee. At the same time, B's right hand attacks A's head (Fig. 8-17). B then turns to the left, causing A to fall (Fig. 8-18).

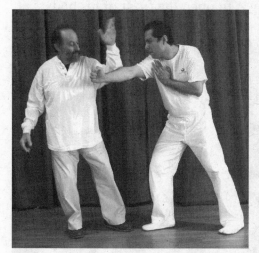

Fig. 8-16

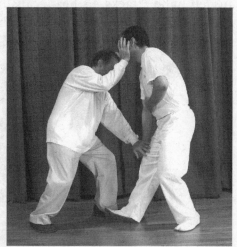

Fig. 8-17

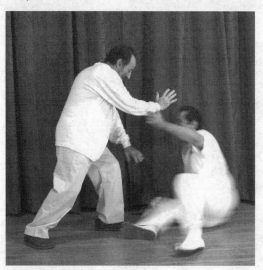

Fig. 8-18

"PUNCH"

B stands with feet naturally apart in a neutral 50-50 stance. Attacker *A* steps forward with his right foot and tries to grab *B*'s shirt with both hands. As *A* moves toward *B*, *B* steps back with his left foot, turning to the left, arms pointing downward. At the same time, *B*'s right shoulder rolls off *A*'s attack (Fig. 8-19). *B* then turns his body to the right and makes a crescent step with his right foot. At the same time, *B*'s arms circle upward and to the right, parrying *A*'s arms. *B* steps forward with his left foot, and his left hand attacks *A*'s head, causing *A* to open the front of his body (Fig. 8-20). *B* then punches *A* with his right hand (Fig. 8-21).

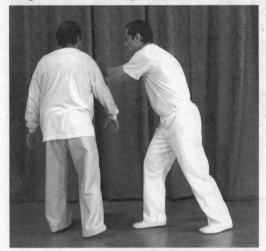

Fig. 8-19

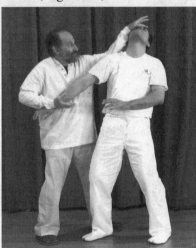

Fig. 8-20

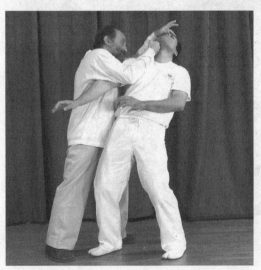

Fig. 8-21

"FIST UNDER ELBOW"

B stands with feet naturally apart in a neutral 50-50 stance. Attacker A steps forward with his left foot and punches B with his left hand. As the punching hand moves toward B, he sidesteps with his left foot, thereby avoiding getting hit. At the same time B slides his left hand along the outside the forearm of A's punching hand (Fig. 8-22). Next, B steps with his right foot, shifts his weight onto that foot, and covers A's left elbow with his right palm (to prevent A from attacking with his elbow) (Fig. 8-23).

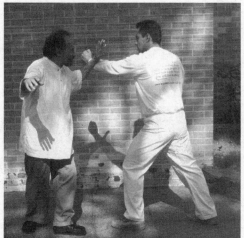

Fig. 8-22

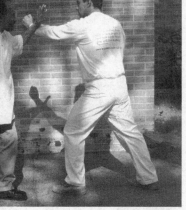

Fig. 8-23

Then B turns to the right and stabs A's neck with the finger tips of his left hand (Fig. 8-24) and can kick A with his left foot (not shown).

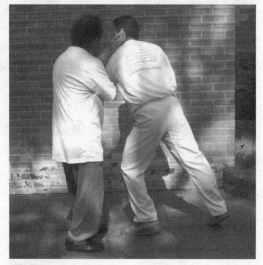

Fig. 8-24

"Golden Cock Stands on One Leg"

B stands with feet naturally apart in a neutral 50-50 stance. Attacker *A* steps forward with his right foot and punches *B* with his right hand. As the punch moves toward *B*, he shifts his weight onto his left foot, thereby avoiding getting hit. At the same time *B* *slides* his right hand along the outside the forearm of *A*'s punching hand (Fig. 8-25), and *B* lifts his left knee and strikes *A*'s abdomen with it (Fig. 8-26).

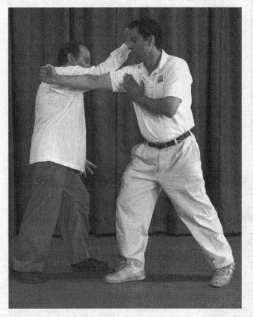

Fig. 8-25

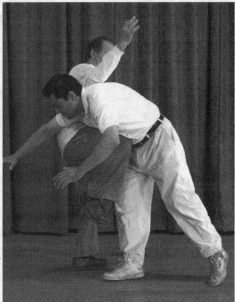

Fig. 8-26

"Fair Lady Works Shuttles"

B stands with feet naturally apart in a neutral 50-50 stance. Attacker A steps forward with his right foot and punches B with his right hand. As the punch moves toward B, he shifts his weight onto his right foot, turns his body to the right and his left foot inward, and interposes his left forearm outside of and perpendicular to the forearm of A's punching hand, thereby avoiding getting hit (Fig. 8-27). Then B shifts his weight onto his left foot and rotates clockwise, rolling his back on A's back (Fig. 8-28). When B has rotated behind A, he strikes A's head and kidneys (Fig. 8-29). Then B brings his right forearm to A's neck and rotates counterclockwise, bringing A down to the ground (Figs. 8-30, 8-31, and 8-32).

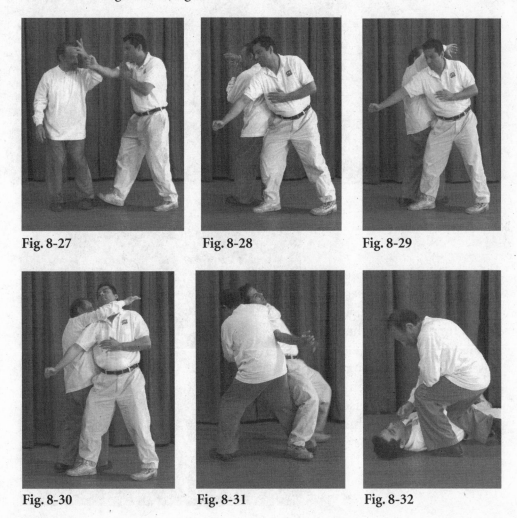

Fig. 8-27   Fig. 8-28   Fig. 8-29

Fig. 8-30   Fig. 8-31   Fig. 8-32

"Step Back to Ride the Tiger"

B stands with feet naturally apart in a neutral 50-50 stance. Attacker A steps forward with his right foot and grabs B's right wrist with his right hand. B steps diagonally backward with his right foot and shifts his weight onto that foot. This action causes A to be pulled into his double-weighted direction. At the same time B covers A's right wrist with his left hand to

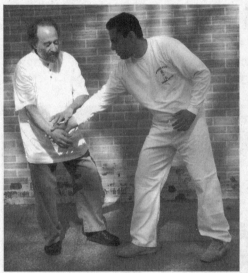

Fig. 8-33

Fig. 8-34

distract A and as a protection in case A's hand releases B's wrist and attacks B (Fig. 8-33). B turns to the right and rotates his right wrist clockwise and escapes through the "gate" (Fig. 8-34). Then B turns his body clockwise, striking A's face with his right hand (Fig. 8-35).

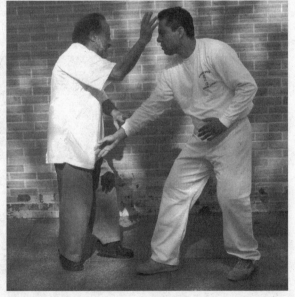

Fig. 8-35

"BEND THE BOW TO SHOOT THE TIGER"

B stands with feet naturally apart in a neutral 50-50 stance. Attacker *A* steps forward with his right foot and tries to push *B* with both hands. As *A* moves toward *B*, *B* steps forward with his right foot, turning to the right, arms pointing downward (Fig. 8-36). At the same time, *B*'s left shoulder rolls off *A*'s attack. *B* then turns his body to the left, circles *A*'s arms downward, outward, and then upward (Fig. 8-37). Then, as *B* turns

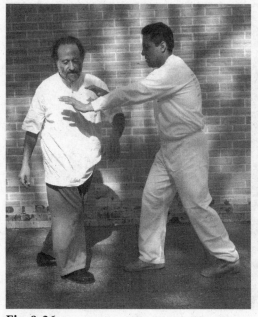

Fig. 8-36

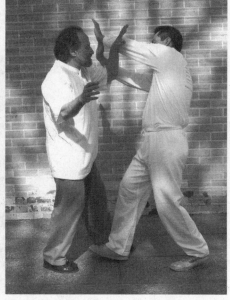

Fig. 8-37

to the left, his right hand attacks *A*'s head (Fig. 8-38), and as *B* turns to the right, his left hand attacks *A*'s body (Fig. 8-39). This application is almost the mirror image of that of "Punch."

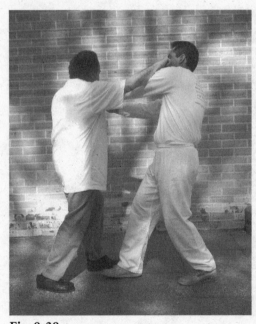 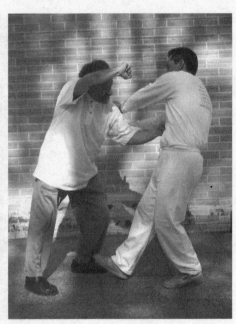

Fig. 8-38   **Fig. 8-39**

9

Taiji as a Martial Art

Taiji was one of the highest fighting arts in China several hundred years ago. Since then, secrecy has resulted in many of the fighting aspects being lost or inaccessible to most students. Even hundreds of years ago, Taiji was not taught until a student was proficient in hard martial-arts styles, so many skills that were not specifically part of Taiji training, per se, were assumed.

The following is an outline of some of the elements required for a rounded martial-arts training. In most cases, many of these elements are missing in most Taiji and other martial-arts teaching. Reliable use of these elements in a self-defense situation requires extensive study under a qualified teacher or succession of teachers. Please do not even attempt to try any of the following elements without a qualified teacher.

KNOWLEDGE OF MODERN SELF-PROTECTION TOOLS

Swords, broadswords, lances, spears, whips, catapults, etc., are outmoded in today's world. Instead, the following tools are either practical to keep in one's home or carried: striking tools (sticks of various lengths from the width of one's palm to 3 feet in length, flashlight, and umbrella),[65] cutting tools (knives of all sizes and everyday items such as keys, a comb, etc.),[66] rope, and projectile tools (handguns, long guns, and shotguns).

---

65. See Masaaki Hatsumi, and Quinton Chambers, *Stick Fighting*, Kdansha International Ltd., New York, 1981, ISBN 0-97011-475-1.
66. See Michael D. Jancich, *Fighting Folders*, VHS, Paladin Press, PO Box 1307, Boulder, CO 80306, ISBN1-58160-093-3.

At the very least, a complete martial art will teach knife, stick, and firearm safety,[67] capabilities, usage, retention, defenses, concealment, and disarms. Periodically, the media tell of untrained citizens who are killed when trying to wrestle a gun from an assailant or because they do not recognize the deadly nature of such tools.

KNOWLEDGE OF QIN NA (GRASPING AND LOCKING TECHNIQUES)

A complete marital-arts training should include joint locks and grasps of skin, hair, sexual organs, throat, bones, muscles, tendons, and nerve centers plus trapping of hands and/or feet by stepping or kneeling on them.

ROLLING AND FALLING

Skills of receiving the ground safely are valuable in daily life, but they are essential as a self-defense escape when tripped or thrown. Rolling can also be used to attack an opponent by kicking or rolling over the attacker or by catapulting an attacker over you, head first, while you roll backwards on top of him. Fear of coming in contact with the ground is very limiting to one's movement options and causes people to stiffen up and become injured when they lose their balance.

DECEPTION

A complete martial art will include skills that cause an opponent to attack on your terms. For example, you can utilize lighting or natural surroundings such as walls, vehicles, or trees to limit the type of attack possible. Or, you can mentally and physically alter an opponent's perception of where you or targets on your body are. Finally, your positioning and movement can lead the opponent to have no expectation or visual awareness of your attack.

DISTANCING

It is crucial to know the distances and angles that put you or your opponent in danger or safety from punches, kicks, sticks, knives (held in a

---

67. See *Home Firearm Safety*, Published By the National Rifle Association of America, 1990.

hand or thrown), firearms of different types (handguns, long guns, shotguns). For example, the effectiveness of each type of firearm depends on its distance from the target. Should someone hold a firearm directly against your back, it is important to know that it is possible to disarm that person relatively easily. But if you are fifteen feet from the attacker, attempting a disarm or escape can be fatal. Training of appropriate methods firearm disarms is necessary. Of course disarming an armed assailant is a bad idea if you have no specialized training or if other conditions are present that might endanger you or another person.

KNOWLEDGE OF LAWS PERTAINING TO USE OF WEAPONS AND DEADLY FORCE

Kevin Harrington, with whom I study Ninjutsu, emphasizes that legal consequences are likely to result from becoming embroiled in a self-defense situation. How witnesses and law-enforcement officers view the situation and what they say in court may not be in your favor even if you were the victim. Moreover, how judges and juries decide the testimony of witnesses and law-enforcement officers will also be critical. In most states, there are very clear legal restrictions on what self-defense tools you are allowed to carry and what you are allowed to do in a self-defense situation.[68] For example, in many states, deadly force is only defensible if your life or that of a loved one is in danger and you are unable to extricate yourself from the situation by running away. Of course, running away may be out of the question in your own house, where there may be no safe place to go, or if running away will put your loved ones in danger.

KNOWLEDGE OF THROWING OBJECTS

A complete marital-arts training should include knowing how to throw dirt, knives, sticks, and other objects. Imaginary objects can be "thrown" as a distraction.

Another valuable skill is the ability to catch a self-defense tool that is thrown to you for your use. Being able to catch or break the fall of a baby can save it from injury or even death.

Also, many people think that knives are effective only at close range. However, knives can, in certain circumstances, be thrown with lethal

---

68. For example, see Karl J. Duff, *Martial Arts & the Law*, Ohara Publications, Burbank. CA, 1985.

effect. Part of training with knives includes knowing whether to hold a knife by its handle or blade when throwing it. This decision is based on the number of half rotations that the knife will undergo at a given distance from the target.

KNOWLEDGE OF STRIKING

A complete martial art will include strikes with hands, feet, elbows, forearms, shoulders, feet, knees, and head. For example, there are many different types of fists for attacking different parts of the body and for producing different effects.

ANATOMY

Knowledge of nerve centers, acupuncture points, muscles, tendons, blood vessels, bones, and organs is important in protecting yourself and also for striking an opponent.

GRAPPLING

According to experienced martial artists, many fights involve grappling and end on the ground. Arts such as wrestling, Jujustu, and Jutaijutsu emphasize dealing with such events.

TAKING PUNCHES

William C.C. Chen is famous for his ability to be unharmed when hit full-force in just about any part of his body. He feels that developing such an ability is important because, whatever your skill level, it is possible that you will be hit during a physical encounter. In some situations, whether getting hit will be debilitating or not can mean the difference between life and death.

HIDING AND EVADING

A complete marital-arts training should include use of natural surroundings and ability to move noiselessly and unnoticed.

KNOWLEDGE OF STRETCHING, NUTRITION, HEALTH, SELF-MASSAGE, AND HEALING

A complete marital-arts training should include principles of optimal diet and of healing injuries.

KNOWLEDGE OF KNOTS; CLIMBING; JUMPING; AND SURVIVAL IN EXTREME HEAT, COLD, AND WATER SUBMERSION

Knowledge of tying knots is not only useful, enjoyable and relaxing but improves dexterity, concentration, and ability to visualize patterns. The kind of coordination of all parts of the body (or lack of it), when brought into play while tying knots, helps to make you aware of the degree to which you have (or have not) incorporated Taiji principles into modalities other than the form. Of course, there is a whole dimension of the use of rope in survival and self-defense applications.

Some other skills are knowledge of specialized breathing to reduce the harmful effects of very hot or cold conditions, the ability to swim with hands and feet tied, the ability to climb steep and smooth walls, knowledge of first aid, and the ability to use sun, moon, stars, and natural surroundings for not getting lost or finding your direction when lost.

KNOWING HOW TO PROTECT YOURSELF FROM CRIME

Protecting yourself in the dojo is not the same as at home, outside, or in your car.[69] Such things as, for example, leaving ample distance between your car and the one in front of you can mean the difference between becoming involved in an accident or not. For example, if your car is hit from behind, it can be launched forward into the car in front of you. Leaving ample space in front can also provide room to escape should a self-defense situation arise.

---

69. For example, see Ira A. Lipman, *How to Protect Yourself from Crime*, Contemporary Books, Chicago, IL, 1989.

Utilizing Creativity in Dealing with Self-Defense Situations

Much self-defense training inculcates preconceived techniques, which may work in some situations. But in other situations, such responses may be worse than those of an untrained person. Higher systems martial-arts training develop the ability to bring inborn creativity to bear in a self-defense situation. The following story illustrates such a creative response to an attack.

Shortly after I started studying Taiji in 1970, I was stuck in a very bad traffic jam in Lower Manhattan. A nearby truck driver started repetitively blasting his air horn. I (stupidly) yelled to him, "Shut up, you big baby." The truck driver instantly jumped out of his truck, bounded toward me, and started to strangle me. Not having learned any self-defense at all, I started to close the window on his arms and began to drive forward toward the next car. The attacker let go, realizing that his arms would get caught in the window and that he might be dragged forward by my car.

Over the years, I have thought about that situation. Of course, I realize the importance of not interacting with other drivers, especially when they are angry to begin with. I have learned to leave a large enough distance between my car and the next to be able to go around that car. I have learned that my unconventional "self-defense" response was creative and solved the problem effectively. The only physical damage I suffered was a bruised neck.

Had I, for example, used a knife to cut my attacker's wrist, he also would have let go. However, my car and clothing would have been drenched in blood. Further, I might have been brought up on criminal charges, or a civil suit might have been brought against me. There is no telling how witnesses might have seen the situation, and they might have testified that *I* was the attacker. Or, the man's friends or family members might have taken reprisal. What if the truck driver had a gun and then used it? Also, if my use of a knife had resulted in the truck driver's death, I would have had to live with having unnecessarily killed a man.

Conclusion

The fact that some of the above facets are *implicit* in Taiji training indicates that they may have been explicitly taught in the past. But without the explicit training, there is little expectation that even the most diligent

Taiji student will be able to apply these facets in a self-defense situation. At least, those lacking explicit training of the elements alluded to in this chapter—and those who study Taiji *primarily* for health and self-development—are more aware and more coordinated, making them less likely to be attacked. They are also more supple and in better physical condition and are, therefore, less susceptible to injury. One would also hope that they are able to avoid and/or run away from a physically threatening situation before self-defense is required.

10

Some Comments About Professor Zheng Manqing

I started Taiji as a beginner with Zheng Manqing (1902–1975) in April, 1970, and continued studying with him until his death. Zheng had come to the United States in the early 1960s to sell his paintings for which he was famous. While here, he was invited to teach a Taiji class to a small group. Zheng stayed to teach an ongoing class. That class drew martial artists such as Lou Kleinsmith, a Judo and Aikido expert; Herman Kauz, a world-class-champion Karate and Judo master who was on the Hawaiian Judo team the year that Hawaii beat Japan; Stanley Israel, who ran a Judo school with Herman Kauz; and Mort Raphael, a Judo expert.

These martial artists were looking for another level of their training that would enable them to do martial arts with a minimum of brute strength. After touching hands with Zheng, they felt that they had encountered the kind of "softness" they were seeking. As Stanley Israel said, "Lou Kleinsmith told me that I must experience the 'Old Man' with whom he had been studying. As soon as I touched hands with Zheng, I knew that he had control of my balance. I decided to study with him right then."

There were also other unusually talented people who became part of the core of an expanding school taught by Prof. Zheng: Ed Young, a highly accomplished artist and illustrator; Maggie Newman, a Kabuki expert and teacher; and Tam Gibbs, a serious student of Asian culture and language.

Zheng was faced with a number of challenging issues. One issue was that he did not speak English and had to communicate through an interpreter or by non-verbal signals. Another issue was that, in the mid 1960s, the main focus of martial artists—and even the general public—was building contractive muscular strength through weight lifting, calisthenics, and isometrics. How was Zheng to teach such subtleties as the powerful expansive strength (*peng jin*), which he had cultivated to a high level, when that kind of strength was antithetical to the strength to which his students were habituated?

The logical route was to teach his students to empty all muscular strength. The emptying of contractive muscular tension is fundamental to Taiji and is called *song*. Analogously, the emptying of mental preconceptions is the basis of Daoism and Buddhism. Thus, Zheng was forming a dual foundation for the development of true physical and mental mastery of Taiji. Zheng also knew that he was getting on in years. With Zheng laying down the right foundation, his students would later be able to continue their studies with the growing number of masters who were emigrating from China and other Asian countries to the United States.

On several occasions, Zheng talked about his not being around for long. On one occasion, he said, "When Confucius was my age, he had only one year to live." On another occasion, Zheng called the whole school together. We all sat on the floor around Zheng while he pointed, in turn, to six senior students, Tam Gibbs, Stanley Israel, Lou Kleinsmith, Maggie Newman, Mort Raphael, and Ed Young (listed here in alphabetical order). Herman Kauz, who was also a senior student of Zheng, had previously left to start his own Taiji school in New York City. "These six," Zheng said, "are equivalent to me. If anything happens to me, these six will carry on in my place." He died a few years afterward.

In his last year of life, Zheng's availability to us suddenly increased. He started teaching courses in advanced form correction, sword correction, push-hands, meditation, Confucius, and Lao Tzu. He taught these courses formally, encouraging questions and answering them through two interpreters, Tam Gibbs and Ed Young, both of whom were very close to Zheng and fluent in Mandarin, Zheng's native dialect.

Zheng originally taught Taiji at the T'ai Chi Ch'uan Association, located at 211 Canal Street in Chinatown, New York City. In spring, 1971, Lou Kleinsmith and Stanley Israel found a new location for the school around the corner, at 87 Bowery, in Chinatown, New York City. Zheng named the school *Shr Jung Center for Culture and the Arts* (*Shr Jung* loosely means being at the right place at the right time). A number of students worked to change what was an industrial loft into an inviting, spacious, well-lit studio with polished hardwood floors and brick walls.

After Zheng's death, the school continued under the direction of the senior students, assisted by students of the next echelon, including me; I had been assisting since 1973, with Zheng's permission (his permission is a separate story, which is accounted in Chapter 13, "Further Development Through Teaching Taiji").

Eventually the senior students went their own separate ways and formed their own schools. At present, Lou Kleinsmith, Tam Gibbs, and Stanley Israel are no longer alive. Maggie Newman and Ed Young each have their own following of many devoted students.

Meanwhile, others who knew Taiji disparaged Zheng's ability or, at least, that of his students. Even now, I frequently hear it said that Zheng Manqing removed the quan (Ch'uan, or martial aspect) from Taijiquan. Zheng's teacher, Yang Cheng-fu (1883–1936), grandson of the legendary Yang Lu-chan (1799–1872), was a famous martial artist who successfully accepted many challenges during his lifetime. In fact, he was considered to be one of the top ten martial artists of the twentieth century. Allegedly, either Zheng did not possess the knowledge to teach his students how to achieve martial skill or did not choose to do so. Of course, many of the criticisms of Zheng came (and still come) from those who met or studied under some of his students but never met him. Unfortunately, many of Zheng's New York students attained a high ability to relax but shunned the idea of developing any kind of strength.

Here is my attempt to explain why so many of Zheng's students fail to show him in the best light: From the time I was a student of Zheng's to this day, his students have held him in the highest regard. This reverence is understandable considering the subtlety and high level of Zheng's skill and his talents beyond those in Taiji. After Zheng's death, many of his students had such reverence for him that they tried to collectively piece together what he had taught rather than seek out new teachers who might set them on a new and, in their view, contradictory and false path. By staying together, they failed to recognize that they had been mainly taught to relax because of (a) their own inability to understand what they were being taught, (b) Zheng's English limitations, and (c) Zheng's death at an early level of their development. They were not yet taught how to be strong because they were not yet ready.

I remember one student asking Zheng the following question: "I can't deal with someone who is very stiff and strong. I can't even deal with my wife's push, and she's not a strong person! Why?" Zheng's answer was simply, "You are not yet ready to deal with strength at your level." From this answer, many students concluded that if they practiced relaxing long enough, they would be able to deal with strength. They didn't recognize that there was a higher level of training yet to come, which involved becoming strong (as in *correct strength*).

Some students actually thought that solely doing the form in a relaxed manner for a number of years without any martial training would make them impervious to any attack. Of course, without any martial training, almost everyone does the same thing when attacked: shields his head with his arms, closes his eyes, and turns away from the attack, exposing his neck and becoming totally defenseless! When I studied under William C.C. Chen, he spent much class time giving us exercises to "deprogram" the turning-away-from-danger response. To this end, Chen would have students pair off and hold a boxing glove lightly in each hand. We would simultaneously tap each other's face with the pillow-like gloves so that we could get hit without flinching or even closing our eyes unless we needed to protect them. Even though we knew we would not get hurt, it still took us a while to "deprogram." So much for being impervious to a real attack without having been exposed to any self-defense training!

Stanley Israel, with his strong martial arts background, was able to absorb much of what Zheng had to teach and saw where it was leading. After Zheng's death, Israel started to teach his own and some of Zheng's remaining students how to achieve the next level, correct strength.

As a first-time visitor to Israel's weekly push-hands class in 1992, I was confronted by a group of men and women for whom my "softness" was useless. I touched hands with one of Israel's students, Mario Napoli, who moved me around with ease. When I complained to Napoli that he was using strength, he replied, "I can be soft too, but if your softness is so good, how come you can't move me?" Right then, I decided that there was more for me to learn, and I came to essentially every Sunday-night push-hands session for the next five years. These two-hour, non-stop sessions were grueling, with very strong people doing their best to be rooted and to uproot me. During summer months, I brought along extra tee shirts to change into and a plastic bag for the sweat-drenched shirts that I successively shed. Gradually, I developed a moderate amount of strength—not the awkward strength of muscular contraction but truly unified, expansive peng. The idea was that "relax" was not an end in itself but a necessary (but not sufficient) condition for developing the true strength of Taijiquan.

Napoli went on to win the all-China competition in push-hands—no small achievement!

In some Taiji circles, the word *strength* is used disparagingly. The confusion arises because there are *two* kinds of strength, described as correct/incorrect, expansive/contractive, and unified/awkward (see Chapter 1). The elusiveness of the difference between the two types of strength is compounded by the lack of any clear explanations of how to experience and cultivate correct strength. Some teachers just say "don't use strength." The result is that their students are afraid to exert any force during push-hands, let their arms collapse, and become righteously indignant when anyone pushes them with more than the legendary "four ounces," which really only applies to the neutralization force—*not to the push*. Zheng made it clear that strength is something to be developed—not force that comes from "tensing of all the muscles" but "tenacious strength."[70] In the words of Stanley Israel, "Taijiquan is a martial art. How can there be a martial art that does not use strength? Of course you need to develop strength, but it must be the right kind."

---

70. See Cheng Man-ch'ing, *T'ai Chi Ch'uan: A Simplified Method of Calisthenics for Health & Self Defense*, North Atlantic Books, Berkeley, CA, 1981, pp. 46–47.

11

Health, Self-Massage, and Healing

HEALTH BENEFITS OF DOING TAIJI

Changes in Conceptual Framework

One of the main differences between Taiji and some other exercises is the engagement of the mind. If you visit a fitness club, you will see rows of people on exercise bikes and treadmills, distracting themselves from the boring nature of what they are doing by watching television, listening to music, and reading magazines—sometimes all at the same time. Most patrons of fitness clubs are interested solely in attaining muscular strength and cardio-vascular fitness and disregard all the other criteria that a Taiji player would consider important for fitness.

Many of the benefits of Taiji stem not only from the immediate changes that occur during practice but also from repeatedly reviewing the principles in your mind and observing whether or not you are manifesting them. These ways of thinking and acting can then be applied even when not practicing Taiji movements per se. For example, if you practice Taiji for any length of time, you will find that, in daily life, you will experience a greater degree of inner calm, self-awareness, balance, and coordination. When outer conditions are anxiety provoking, there is a natural tendency for Taiji practitioners to sink their weight and breathe in a beneficial manner.

The Effects of Muscular Extension and
Passive Movement on the Acidity of the Body

Correct practice of Taiji movement involves using muscles in a different way from that during other movement or exercise; namely, we are using muscular extension instead of muscular contraction. Also, there is a lot of passive movement rather than active movement. In passive movement, gravity, linear momentum, rotational momentum, and the centrifugal effects of circular movements cause muscles to move without their doing so actively.

All this means that while doing Taiji, instead of producing lactic acid (as in ordinary exercise), we are actually getting rid of it. Lactic acid is normally difficult to get rid of, and while it is present, constitutes an acid state in the body, irritates muscles, and produces fatigue. Lactic acid is eventually converted into water and carbon dioxide, which is also acidic (carbonic acid). But carbon dioxide is readily eliminated via the lungs.

AWARENESS OF THE EFFECTS OF OUR
ACTIONS AND OF EXTERNAL INFLUENCES

Some people will repeat actions that are damaging to themselves and continue to do so for a long time because they do not connect these actions with the harm done by them. For example, when eating, do you notice only the effect of food on the tongue and teeth, or do you also notice the effect on the stomach and the rest of the body while you are eating and afterward? When doing exercise, are you merely following the hype of the latest fad and ignoring its damaging effects on your body?

Unfortunately, some of the ill effects of our actions do not occur instantaneously but from hours to years later. This delay plus the large number of things we say, do, and consume makes it very difficult to unscramble the effects of our actions. For example, decades ago, I used to drink brewed, caffeinated coffee and loved it. One day, a friend asked me, "Did you ever notice how rotten you feel 5 or 6 hours after you drink a cup of coffee." I realized that I had been feeling that way but never connected it with drinking coffee. I promptly stopped drinking coffee except for decaffeinated coffee and do not experience that "rotten" feeling unless someone substitutes regular coffee for decaffeinated coffee; then, I realize it 5 or 6 hours later. Similarly, people with wrong alignment of their knees and ankles almost never associate the resulting chronic or acute harm with how they are using their bodies. There are many other examples having to do with body usage, intake of food and drink, our thoughts, and what we say.

One of the purposes of doing Taiji and/or meditative stretching daily is to begin associating an anomaly in how your body feels on a given day with what you subjected your body to yesterday and the day before—both positive and negative. Some examples are food, pharmaceuticals, artificial flavor, sugar, thoughts, sleep, interactions with others, exercise, sex, bodily usage, and even the phases of the moon. When you stretch on a daily basis, such a pervasive awareness builds.

When I was working on my Ph.D. thesis, I was using radioactive materials, 1000 °C ovens, explosive gasses, highly corrosive acids, vacuum pumps containing liquid mercury, and very expensive equipment. Being less than at my best on a given day could easily result in serious injury to myself, damage to valuable equipment, and a failure of my experiment. On days when I did not feel right, I didn't work on my thesis but took the day off. Doing so may have saved my life.

Zheng Manqing's Criteria for the Frequency of Sexual Activity

The following are my notes from one of Professor Zheng's lectures in 1973:

"There is a big difference between the east and west, and there is another big difference between the ancient- and modern-Chinese points of view. I am most familiar with the ancients.

"There is big desire: sex and eating, and small desire: money, power, and having many women. If the big desire turns into lust, then we will gorge ourselves. The distinction is that the big desire is based on necessity and the preservation of the species.

"In ancient times, boys reached puberty at 16 years of age and girls at 14 years of age. Westerners are about one year ahead of Chinese [in sexual development when both are] at 6 years of age.

"If you expect to live for 120 years, you must heed the following:

Age in Years	Time for Sexual Renewal
16	1 week
24	2 weeks
32	3 weeks
40	40 days
50	infinite

"If you borrow from the bank every day, there will come a time when you will be bankrupt. All animals have a season when they get in heat; humans can mess up at any time. Rein in your passions. Practicing Taiji will help. When you have a desire to have sexual intercourse, do your best to cut down. Don't let your passions run away."

I remember a student asking Zheng if the criteria applied to both males and females. Zheng said it only applied to males.

Life Spans of Taiji Practitioners

Table 11-1 lists the life spans of thirty-two of some of the famous Taiji masters, born over 100 years ago, listed in order of chronology of birth, with names spelled in Wade-Giles Romanization[71] to facilitate Internet searching.

The median and average ages are both about 72 years, which may seem low but are actually quite high considering conditions in China in the 1700s, 1800s, and early 1900s (none on the list was born past 1906). Of the masters listed above, Chen You–long and Yang Cheng-fu had the shortest life spans (53 years), and Liang Tung-tsai (T. T. Liang) and Lu Dian-chen had the longest (102 and 105 years, respectively). It is interesting to note that in his later years, Yang Cheng-fu was not a man of moderation. According to Zheng Manqing, Yang would sometimes feast for a whole week. He become so obese that he could not do "Golden Cock Stands on One Leg." Evidently some of these masters felt themselves to be invincible and were prone to indulge in excesses of food and wine,[72] which shortened their lives.

BACK OR KNEE PAIN

Dealing with Back Problems

I developed a severe curvature of the spine in my mid-twenties. I went to doctors for back pain, but none even touched my back or examined at its shape. Instead, they ordered tests, which revealed that my kidney function was normal. The pain was blamed on various things such as "having too much sex"! When I started studying movement arts, each teacher immediately noticed the problem and promised to deal with it. Taiji, Shiatsu, strengthening exercises, chiropractic, meditation, and visualization all had

---

71. The distinctions between Wade-Giles and pinyin are discussed in Ch. 12.
72. Chinese wine has about 40% alcohol, twice as much as fortified European and American wines.

Table 11-1. Life spans of some famous Taiji practitioners born over one-hundred years ago, listed in order of birth date.

Name	Birth–Death Dates	Life Span in Years
Chen Chang–hsing	1771–1853	82
Chen Ching–ping	1795–1868	73
Yang Lu–ch'an	1799–1872	73
Chen Che–sang	1809–1865	56
Chen Chung–san	1809–1871	62
Wu Yu–hsiang	1812–1880	68
Lee I–yu	1833–1892	59
Yang Pan–hou	1837–1892	55
Yang Chien–hou	1839–1917	78
Kuo Wei–jin	1849–1920	59
Ch'en P'in–san	1849–1929	80
Sun Lu–t'ang	1860–1932	72
Yang Sou–hou	1862–1930	68
Wu Chien–chuan	1870–1942	72
Yang Zhao–pen	1872–1930	58
Chen You–long	1875–1928	53
Hou Yao–yu	1877–1935	58
Hsu Yu–sang	1878–1945	66
Fu Chen–sung	1881–1953	72
Chen Wei–Ming	1881–1958	77
Yang Cheng–fu	1883–1936	53
Choy Heng–peng	1886–1957	71
Lu Dian-chen	1886–1991	105
Chen Fa–kor	1887–1957	70
Cui Yi–shi	1890–1970	80
Wu Meng-xia	1890–1970	80
Kuo Lien–ying	1891–1984	93
Tung Ying-chieh	1898–1961	63
Chen Pan–lin	1900–1967	67
Cheng Man–ch'ing	1900–1975	75
Liang Tung–tsai (T.T. Liang)	1900–2002	102
Hu Yuen–chou	1906–1997	91

their benefits, but none of these modalities seemed to help much. The pain was so intense that during the course of each day, I would have to find a place to lie on my back for several minutes to alleviate the pain. It was not until I studied Kinetic Awareness with Elaine Summers that I started to understand the factors involved and how to reverse or at least arrest them.

One of the key things Summers taught me was to gain mobility of my spine through lying on my back on from one to five balls, isolating each segment of my spine and moving it very slowly in all directions. The other key for dealing with the curvature of my spine was applying muscular extension, a concept she taught me.

Essentially, when there is any abnormal forward curvature of the spine, the muscles in the back become stretched and traumatized. They are in an almost constant state of pain. Moreover, because of the leverage required, they have to exert inordinately large contractive forces for extended periods of time to straighten the curvature. Because muscular contraction can only be sustained for short periods of time, the back muscles have only one choice, namely, to relax and let themselves be stretched even more. Thus, the process is cyclic, and the spine becomes increasingly curved.

The only solution to this vicious cycle that I have found (other than wearing a brace) that works is to use muscular extension of the muscles on the front (interior aspect) of the spine for supporting the back (taught to me by Summers). Muscular extension can be sustained much longer than muscular contraction, so the back muscles can relax for extended periods of time, allowing blood and qi to penetrate.

Knee Pain

It is not uncommon for Taiji practitioners to experience knee pain. The problem is that such pain can have many causes and may even have nothing to do with the knee, itself. The pain can result from overuse of leg muscles, incorrect alignment of the knees, or hyperextending the knees (beginning Taiji players are taught not to hyperextend any part of the body). If the pain comes from overuse, the simple answer is not to sink into stances until the problem is gone. If the pain comes from incorrect alignment (discussed in detail in prior books of mine[73] and in abbreviated form in Chapter 5 of this book under the admonition, "The knee should not go past the toe"), then that alignment should be corrected. It is my experience that the pain stemming from habitual hyperextension of the knees often disappears soon after the habit is broken.

Knee pain is often diagnosed as tendonitis of the tendons that attach to the patella (knee cap) and treated with physiotherapy. Sometimes the physiotherapy extends into years with no success.

I have found that students of mine who complain of knee pain often are experiencing reflected pain from the quadriceps or calf muscles. The site of pain can be revealed by methodically palpating all the musculature above and below the knee. The muscles and tendons on the inside of the thigh are the most common ones to cause knee pain. Therapy consists of (1) staying away from stressful movement or positions that increase the pain and (2) professional or self-massage of the affected muscles and/or tendons.

Often, knee pain is diagnosed as stemming from a torn meniscus, and surgery is suggested. Before submitting to surgery, it is probably a good idea to seek second and third opinions of sports trainers or M.D.'s.

When the pain results from incorrect alignment, physiotherapy, in my view, is not very effective. The prevailing medical misconception is that incorrect alignment results from an imbalance of the muscles, and therapy consists in strengthening the weaker muscles. The reason that this approach is futile is that its premise involves a reversal of cause and effect. Actually, the weaker muscles result from the lack of use *because of* the incorrect alignment. The cause of incorrect alignment is a faulty conception of the correct relationship of the bones of the legs, which can only be corrected by learning the correct relationship and overcoming life-long habits over time by practicing the correct way.

SELF-MASSAGE

The advantages of doing self-massage are that you can attend to a problem immediately, you remain independent, and you learn about your body. For parts of the body that are easy to reach such as hands, arms, and thighs, self-massage simply consists of using the fingers knuckles, and/or elbows to apply movement and pressure of appropriate degree to the affected region(s). It is a good idea to massage a muscle in its most relaxed state. When it comes to massaging one's own back, special techniques need to be employed. The following are a number of alternative ways of doing massage of various parts of the body.

---

73. Robert Chuckrow, *Tai Chi Walking*, YMAA Publication Center, Boston, MA, 2002, pp.; Robert Chuckrow, *The Tai Chi Book*, YMAA Publication Center, Boston, MA, 1998, pp.

Self-Massage of Head

Massage of the head has many benefits including relaxing the jaw and eyes and stimulating flow of blood, oxygen, and qi to the eyes, teeth, lymph nodes, hair follicles, and brain. I prefer to massage my head while lying on the floor on my back, with a pillow under my head, but a head massage can also be done while standing or sitting.

1. Start by massaging the temples with the tips of the fingers (Fig. 11-1).
2. Next, massage the scalp with the tips of the fingers (Fig. 11-2).
3. Massage the jaw muscles (between the eyes and ears) with the tips of the fingers (Fig. 11-3).
4. Massage the jaw muscles (at the end of the jaw) with the tips of the fingers (Fig. 11-4).
5. Massage the jaw bone with the tips of the thumbs (Fig. 11-5).
6. Cautiously and gently massage the glands underneath the jaw by hooking the tips of the thumbs under the jaws (Fig. 11-6).
7. Massage the roots of the lower teeth (Fig. 11-7).
8. Massage the roots of the upper teeth (Fig. 11-8).
9. Massage the musculature under the cheekbones by using the tips of the thumbs (Fig. 11-9).
10. Massage the bony tissue on the sides of the nose by using the tips of the fingers (Fig. 11-10).

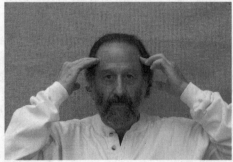

Fig. 11-1.

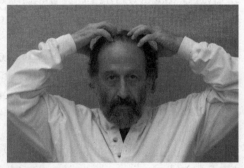

Fig. 11-2.

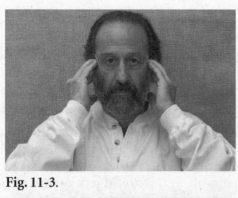

Fig. 11-3.

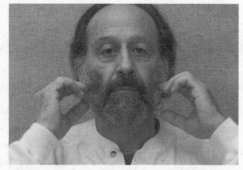

Fig. 11-4.

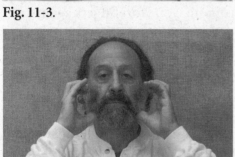

Fig. 11-5.

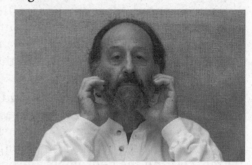

Fig. 11-6.

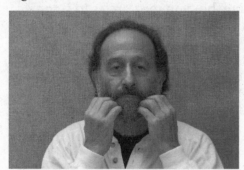

Fig. 11-7.

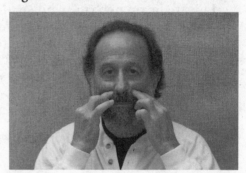

Fig. 11-8.

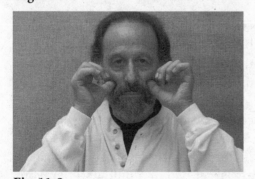

Fig. 11-9.

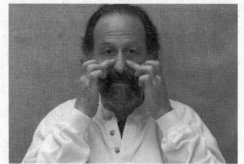

Fig. 11-10.

11. Massage the erector muscles on the sides of the neck (Fig. 11-11).

12. Massage the skin on the back and sides of the neck by rolling it between the thumb and fingers (Fig. 11-12).

13. Massage the ears (Fig. 11-13).

14. Massage the ear canals by inserting the little fingers and jiggling them (Fig. 11-14).

15. When I was a beginning student under Zheng Manqing, he made a special point of showing me a massage for the eyes. The massage does not actually involve any pressure on the eyes but, rather, on the bony ridges of the eye sockets. Start by propping your forefingers against your forehead. Place the first joints (near the nail) of your thumb against the outside corners of your eyes (Fig. 11-15). Move the thumb joints inward along the top of the ridges of the eye sockets and then out along the bottoms in a continuous circling motion. Repeat for a total of 36 times.

16. This exercise is called *palming* and is considered to be the most important exercise for relaxing your eyes (Fig. 11-16). We tend to misuse and over use our eyes because of the pace of our modern society and the use of electricity to extend the length of the day. So resting the eye muscles and the neurological processing of images is highly beneficial.

    I like to lie on my back while palming, but you may prefer to sit or stand. Start by rubbing your palms together to develop warmth and qi. Place your palms over your eyes to create dark warm caves for your eyes. Allow warmth to develop and enjoy the darkness and absence of need to receive or process visual sense data. While the eyes rest and are bathed in warmth, allow them to relax and relinquish the necessity to seek out images. Think of the eyes as pools of liquid resting in the eye sockets.

Self-Massage of Back

One way of massaging back muscles is to use one or more balls under your back while lying on the floor on your back. I find that 4- and 5-inch-diameter rubber or plastic air-filled balls work best (the larger ball goes under your head). Such balls are found in toy or sporting-goods stores. First lie on your back without the balls until a state of deep relaxation is achieved. Then, using your hands, place one or more balls under your back. If you use two balls, they can go along your spine. If you use a single ball, it can go anywhere on your back including under a shoulder. Make sure to support your head with a slightly larger ball or a pillow so that your cervical spine is in a neutral alignment. Relax and give in to gravity,

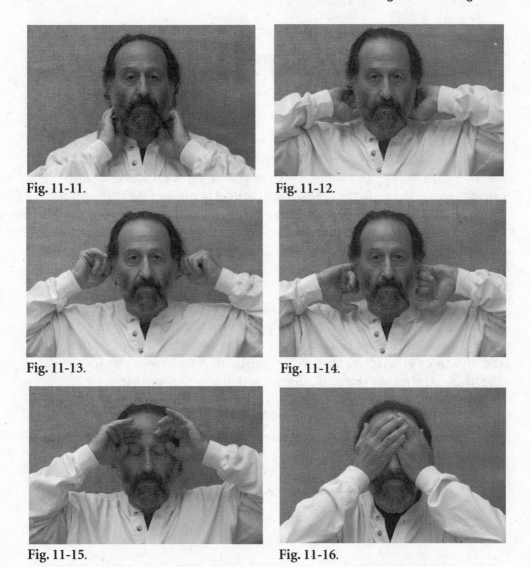

Fig. 11-11.

Fig. 11-12.

Fig. 11-13.

Fig. 11-14.

Fig. 11-15.

Fig. 11-16.

making slight, slow, gentle movements of the spine in all directions. Then slowly roll up or down to allow the pressure of the ball(s) to penetrate each region in succession. If there is any pain, do not remain in that position. When you are finished, remove the ball(s) and lie on your back awhile, letting the whole body give in to gravity as much as possible. When you feel ready to get up, roll over onto one side, and come up slowly, using your hands and arms rather than the muscles around the spine.

I usually take a rubber softball with me whenever I drive my car. I place the ball between my back and the seat as I drive.

Some Exercises for the Back

Figures 11-17 through 11-25 show beneficial stretches for the back (taught to me by Elaine Summers). I constructed the foam-topped hassock shown specifically for this exercise, but other items can be used such as a bed, a couch, or an, under-inflated ball.

Caution: *Please consult a health-care professional before attempting these exercises, which can involve strenuous stretching of the muscles of the back and chest. If you have any doubt that you can do these exercises, do not attempt them! If you do try them, it is essential to proceed very slowly and carefully, and slide off if you experience any pain. The first time you try these exercises it is important to have someone else there to assist you if necessary. After stopping, make certain to rest in a neutral position before placing any stress on the muscles that have been stretched beyond their accustomed range.*

Start out by resting on your back (Fig. 11-17).

After a state of relaxation is achieved, slowly move so that the edge of the hassock under your head is lower on your spine (Fig. 11-18). Relax and give in to gravity, making slight, gentle movements of the spine in all directions. If there is any pain, do not remain in that position.

Then, slowly move your body so that your head moves closer to the floor (Figs. 11-19 and 11-20).

When the top of your head rests on the floor (Fig. 11-21), dwell in that position, letting the whole body give in to gravity as much as possible.

Next, move your body so that the back of your neck rests on the floor (Fig. 11-22), and dwell in that position, letting the whole body give in to gravity as much as possible.

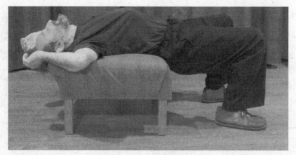

Fig. 11-17.

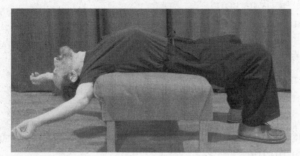

Fig. 11-18.

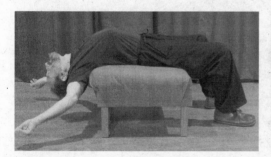

Fig. 11-19.

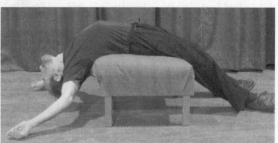

Fig. 11-20.

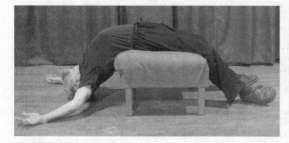

Fig. 11-21.

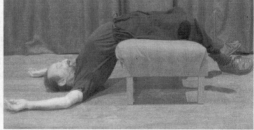

Fig. 11-22.

Next, slide down so that your entire spine rests on the floor (Fig. 11-23), and dwell in that position, letting the whole body give in to gravity as much as possible. There are two ways to slide down: One way is to let the hassock slowly slide away from your body as you gently lower yourself. The other way is to use your arms and legs to push yourself off. When you feel ready to get up, roll over onto one side, and rise slowly, using your hands and arms rather than the muscles around the spine.

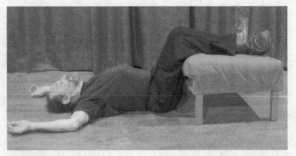

Fig. 11-23.

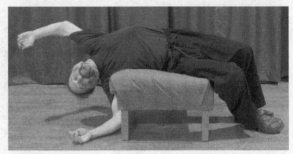

Fig. 11-24.

Most stretching exercises for the spine involve forward and backward stretching but not sideways stretching. A hassock provides an opportunity to stretch the spine sideways (Fig. 11-24).

Then rest on your back on the hassock until you are ready to do the other side

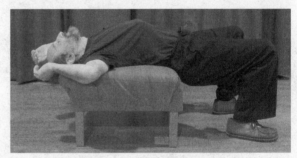

Fig. 11-25.

(Fig. 11-25). After doing the other side, rest on your back on the hassock until you are ready to rise to standing or sitting. When you rise, do so by rolling over onto one side, slowly coming up sideways, using your hands and arms rather than the muscles around the spine.

Self-Massage of Legs

One way of massaging calf or thigh muscles is to lie on the floor on your back or abdomen, respectively, and place a ball under the affected region. Then do small movements that allow the pressure of the ball to penetrate every region. I find that a softball made of dense rubber works best.

Another way to massage a calf muscle is to lie on your back on the floor, with the knee of one leg up. Let the calf of the other leg rest on that knee, doing slow, methodical movements to cover every region of the calf (see Fig. 11-26). To massage the quadriceps, I lie on my back on the floor, with one leg outstretched. Then I use the heel of my other foot to massage the quadriceps of my outstretched leg (see Fig. 11-27). Whatever massage is done on one side should always be repeated on the other.

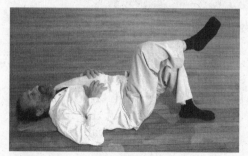
Fig. 11-26. *Self-massage of calf.*

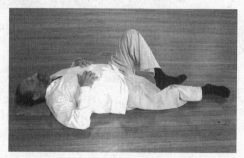
Fig. 11-27. *Self-massage of quadriceps.*

Self-Massage of Feet

Most footwear does not permit the full muscular movement of feet. Unless you walk exclusively during warm weather and on soft ground, you probably will not do much walking barefooted. In most cases, you will need to wear some sort of footwear, which, over any period of time, will inhibit the natural movement of your feet.

Massaging your own feet or having them massaged is very beneficial, especially when you are sick. As illustrated by Fig. 11-28, foot massage can be taught to young children and appreciated by them.

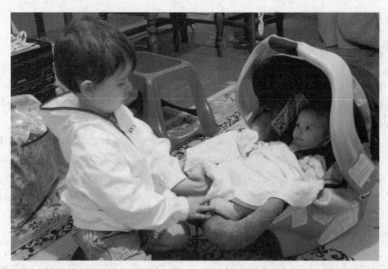

Fig. 11-28. *The author's three-year-old grandson giving his three-month-old sister a foot massage.*

The following foot massage will be of much value in toning the feet:[74]

1. While sitting, lift one foot and let it rest on your thigh. Grab the toes with the opposite hand and rotate the whole foot about the ankle fifteen times in one direction (see Fig. 11-29). Then repeat fifteen times in the other direction.

2. Grab the toes with the opposite hand and rotate the whole toe end of the foot, first in one direction and then in the other direction (see Fig. 11-30).

3. Sitting, bend one knee and lift the foot on that side. Reach under the foot with the opposite hand so that the end of the fifth metatarsal[75] is cradled in the hollow of the palm. Then similarly cradle the first metatarsal in the palm of the other hand. Applying moderate pressure, briskly move the hands toward and away from the body in opposite directions. This action will cause the foot to be twisted back and forth (see Fig. 11-31).

4. Grab the big toe between your thumb and forefinger of the hand opposite the foot and crank the toe in a circle. Crank each toe in turn (see Fig. 11-32).

5. Squeeze the sides of the first joint (near the root of the nail) of the big toe between your thumb and forefinger. Roll the joint back and forth in each direction (see Fig. 11-33). Repeat with each toe in turn.

---

74. This massage routine is reproduced from Robert Chuckrow, *Tai Chi Walking*, YMAA Publication Center, Boston, MA, 2002, pp. 70–72.

75. A metatarsal is a long bone within the foot to which a toe is joined.

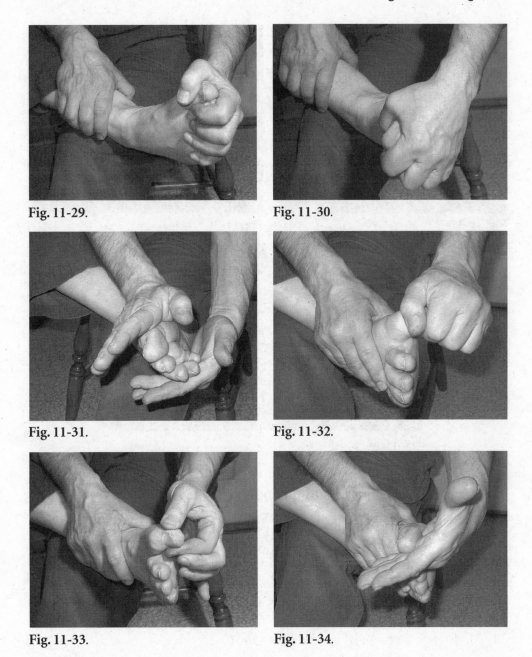

Fig. 11-29.   Fig. 11-30.

Fig. 11-31.   Fig. 11-32.

Fig. 11-33.   Fig. 11-34.

6. Place the outer edge of your extended hand between the big toe and the next. Then massage the space between with a vigorous sawing motion. Repeat for each successive pair of toes (see Fig. 11-34).

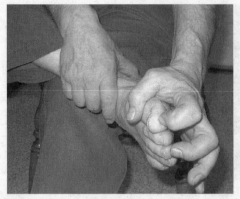

Fig. 11-35.

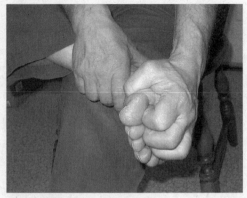

Fig. 11-36.

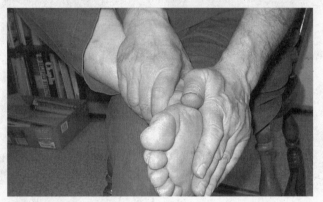

Fig. 11-37

7. Dig the nails of fingers into the tips of the toes (see Fig. 11-35).

8. Dig the nails of fingers into the roots of the toes (see Fig. 11-36).

9. Starting at the inner ankle, briskly rub the palm of the hand across the arch toward the little toe and back. This rub was taught to me by Zeng Manqing, who instructed me to do this rub twenty-one times to each foot (see Fig. 11-37).

10. End by feeling the qi entering the yongquan point ("bubbling well") located on the center of the sole of the foot, just below the ball of the foot.

11–20. Repeat steps 1–10 on the other foot.

Healing

Differences Between American Medicine and Traditional Chinese Medicine.

Western medicine has its roots in the belief that disease is caused by evil spirits entering the body. Treatment originally consisted of driving out the evil spirits by introducing poisons such as mercury or by bleeding. Luis Pasteur (1822–1895) was a scientist working on the question of why wine turned to vinegar (became sick). When Pasteur discovered that bacteria were responsible for diseases of wine, the medical profession decided that human and animal diseases were also caused by bacteria. Thus, the theory that evil spirits caused disease was finally borne out by science. When antibiotics were discovered, the medical profession now had found a way to destroy the evil spirits.

Because the application of science had been found to be so successful in discovering the evil spirits and their destruction, science was applied to other areas of western medicine. Western medicine has thousands of blood tests that can uncover unhealthy states of the body and a very complete knowledge of anatomy, physiology, genetics, and the hormonal system. Also, modern medicine has contributed important knowledge of hygiene and the modes of transmission of diseases.

Unfortunately, modern medicine has two limitations. One limitation is that its knowledge is primarily used as a means of making huge profits for pharmaceutical and health-insurance companies. A consequence of the monetary emphasis is the rejection of knowledge that threatens profits. The other limitation (not unrelated to the first) is that modern medicine does not place enough emphasis on the body's ability to fend off disease through nutrition, lifestyle, and exercise.

A good part of the development of Traditional Chinese Medicine (TCM) originated in the martial arts. When two warriors were embroiled in a life-and-death struggle, and both were too injured to carry on the struggle, the one who could recover first had a distinct advantage. Therefore, martial artists had a strong incentive to become knowledgeable about the healing effects of natural substances. Even though it is rare for today's martial artists to engage in hand-to-hand combat, many martial-arts practitioners have knowledge of herbal and other remedies.

TCM includes highly effective remedies for setting broken bones, stopping internal and external bleeding from strikes and knife wounds, and treatments for trauma to muscles, ligaments and tendons. TCM also is useful in strengthening the immune system and diagnosing and treating a large variety of ailments and diseases.

The main conceptual framework of TCM involves treating disruptions to the flow of qi by the use of herbs and acupuncture. Some of the herbs used in TCM have been known for hundreds of years, others for thousands. Some Chinese remedies are claimed to go back as far as 2,000–3,000 BC. The main part of traditional Chinese medicine is the use of herbs to provide many of the above benefits and others not known outside of Asia such as improving the circulation of qi, balancing yin and yang, and balancing the five elements, namely earth, air, fire, water, and metal. One web site[76] lists over 2,270 different substances used in TCM.

Trial and error certainly was employed in learning the benefits of various herbs. However, over time, some herbalists developed the ability to smell and taste an herb and thereby know what ailments it could benefit. Zheng Manqing is said to have been taught such a skill.

The subject of herbs is one about which many books have been written in all parts of the world and to which many people devote their entire lives. This book cannot even hope to scratch the surface of such a vast subject.

It is my view that the knowledge of both TCM and western medicine, if merged, would be much more effective than either system alone.

Stories About Traditional Chinese Medicine

Story 1. A student came to study Taiji with me who was very sick. She was a woman in her thirties who weighed 80 pounds, had not menstruated in five years, and excreted her food without digesting it. She had been to several western doctors who accused her of being anorexic, which she denied emphatically. However, they had no protocol whatsoever for treating her condition.

I recommended that she see my herbalist/acupuncturist, Zhang Qingcai. After about a year of treatment with TCM, she was digesting her food normally, she had gained thirty pounds, and her menstrual period had returned.

Story 2. A friend who is a guitar virtuoso developed a fungus infection on his fingernails. Over a period of time, his fingernails began to disintegrate. He went to a dermatologist, who prescribed a salve. My friend applied the

---

76. See www.ccat.sas.upenn.edu/~nsivin/mm.html, *Index to Shiu-Ying Hu, An Enumeration of Chinese Materia Medica*, Hong Kong, 1980.

salve for weeks, but his nails became worse. On my advice, he went to Zhang, who prescribed concentrated allicin (one of the active principles in garlic) to be taken internally and swabbed directly on the fingernails. The fungus condition completely disappeared within a few days.

It should be noted that garlic is highly effective in killing not only fungus but also bacteria, viruses, and parasites.

Story 3. Recently, an elderly relative of mine was hospitalized for a possible stroke. When I visited him in the hospital, his face had been shaven. Because of the blood thinners he had been given, the shaving cuts on his face had been bleeding for hours despite the nurses' efforts.

I always carry a vial of Yinan Paiyao, which is a powder that is famous in China for stopping bleeding. I applied the Yinan Paiyao to the cuts, and the bleeding stopped within minutes. The nurses were relieved that I had stopped the bleeding but showed little interest in the remedy that was used.

Note: I advise those who seek an acupuncturist to consider selecting one who is also a herbalist. The reason is that acupuncture is a minor part of TCM, but herbs are a major part. Those practitioners without expertise in herbology will tend to treat everything with acupuncture even if acupuncture is not an effective tool for that condition. "When your only tool is a hammer, everything looks like a nail."

THERAPEUTIC FASTING

This section on fasting, reproduced from the author's book on nutrition[77] and updated for this book, is included for reference purposes only, not because fasting is recommended but because having an understanding of it can help in other areas. Should anyone decide to embark on a fast, the author emphasizes the importance of seeking a competent professional to supervise any fast beyond several days.

Fasting refers to a complete abstinence from everything of nutritive value (but not abstinence from water) for a period of time. A common mistake, even in medical books, is to confuse fasting with starvation. During fasting, the body draws on its reserves in a beneficial manner.

77. Robert Chuckrow, *The Intelligent Dieter's Guide*, Rising Mist Publications, Briarcliff Manor, NY, 1997, Ch. 11 (available from http://www.bestweb.net/~taichi).

Starvation begins when the reserves are exhausted, and if sufficiently prolonged, starvation ends in death.

Because the subject of fasting is vast, anyone considering fasting is encouraged to read at least one of the classical books on the subject.[78, 79, 80, 81, 82, 83] Because some of these books are difficult to find, a search on the Internet for "therapeutic fasting" or "fasting can save your life" should provide information on fasting and those who supervise fasts.

Reasons for Fasting

Most of us are exposed to pesticides; polluted air and water; pharmaceuticals; medical X-rays; nuclear background radiation; improper amounts of sunlight; devitalized foods that are missing essential nutrients and laced with pesticides, artificial colors and flavors; and food eaten in amounts and combinations impossible to properly digest, leading to bacterial decomposition and absorption of incompletely digested proteins. Over time, these factors plus dead tissue throughout our bodies cause inflammation, reduced or unnaturally stepped-up immune-system function, and even tumors. Fasting is a way of reducing or eliminating such factors or to restore health when one is ill.

Benefits of Fasting

The beneficial effects of fasting have been known for thousands of years. Pythagoras (c582–c500 B.C.) is said to have required those who wanted to study with him to fast for forty days beforehand. The Bible mentions fasting numerous times. Benjamin Franklin is reputed to have said, "*The best of all medicines are rest and fasting.*" Zoos fast their predatory animals one or two days a week to extend their life spans and improve their health. Unfortunately, modern medicine disregards fasting and rejects the possibility that it may have any value. One need only fast for a few days to become acquainted with its benefits, which include improved functioning of the brain

---

78. Herbert M. Shelton, *Fasting and Sunbathing*, Dr. Shelton's Health School, San Antonio, TX, 1963.

79. Arnold De Vries, *Therapeutic Fasting*, Chandler Book Co., Los Angeles, CA, 1963. This book is out of print but can be obtained from http://www.soilandhealth.org/copyform.aspx?bookcode=020141.

80. Hereward Carrington, *Fasting for Health and Long Life*, Health Research, Mokelumne Hill, CA, 1953.

81. Herbert M. Shelton, *Fasting Can Save Your Life*, Natural Hygiene Press, Inc., Chicago, IL, 1964.

82. Some of Shelton's writings, possibly in edited form, are available from the American Natural Hygiene Society, P.O. Box 30630, Tampa Fl 33630, 813-855-6607.

83. Paul C. Bragg, *The Miracle of Fasting*, Health Science, Box 15000, Santa Anna, CA 92705, 1975. Perhaps this book is not a classic; nevertheless, it provides much worthwhile information.

and nervous system, rest for the entire digestive tract, and stepped-up elimination of toxins.

During fasting, effects of negative interactions, insufficient intake of water, and overuse of the body are highly amplified. This increased sensitivity affords the opportunity to learn much. Of value is realizing how much eating we do that is not in response to a physiological need for food. When undesirable states of the body subside during fasting, it is possible to generally ascribe them to food. After the fast is broken and foods are introduced into the diet one-by-one, there is an opportunity to unscramble the beneficial, harmful, or addictive effects of substances we ingest. There is also an opportunity to see the beneficial effects of proper food combining for optimal digestion.[84]

As one who has fasted a number of times ranging from one to 28 days, I credit fasting with vastly improving my vision, digestion, clarity of thought, and general health. During a 26-day fast in 1971, among other benefits, a testicular cyst that I had had for decades completely disappeared and never came back.

After a few difficult days of fasting, during which one may be ravenously hungry and weak, interest in food becomes essentially absent, and a marvelous feeling of energy appears. Of course, there may be periods of weakness, nausea, and other unpleasant symptoms caused by heavy toxins that are exiting the body. If the fast is continued, hunger eventually returns to signal a natural end to the fast.

How Fasting Works

The underlying principle of fasting is that when the body is forced to utilize its own reserves, it uses the least essential nutritive material first. Therefore, fat, toxins and undigested nutrients residing in cells, dead cells, and even tumors are eliminated quickly and efficiently. To understand why the body works in this manner, consider that human life has been on this earth for about a million years, but the life forms from which we have evolved go back thousands of millions of years. Over this period, life forms have been periodically exposed to conditions under which there was no food for extended periods of time. Even one extra day of starvation can mean the difference between life and death. The evolutionary pressure on life forms to survive as long as possible without food thus gave rise to the ability to utilize every non-essential part in time of deprivation.

---

84. See Robert Chuckrow, *The Intelligent Dieter's Guide*, Ch. 6 (available from http://www.bestweb.net/~taichi).

Thus, humans have the capacity to utilize the least-needed reserves once deprivation of food extends for even a day. Expired cells (the proportion of which increases with biological age), partially digested proteins in the system, and even tumors all have some nutritive value. It makes sense that, for survival, the body will absorb this morbid material, excrete the toxins therein, and extract anything of nutritive value. The main action of the body is survival in the absence of food, but the secondary effects are a thorough cleansing of the system.

Of course, once the unneeded reserves are exhausted, fasting ends. Now starvation begins, in which essential tissues must be utilized for staying alive. Starvation ends in death. That is why it is of utmost importance for anyone on a long-term fast to distinguish the line between fasting and starvation. When fasting ends, one or both of two things occur. One is the clearing of coating on the tongue. The other is a return of true hunger, which is noticeably absent during the fast. The return of hunger is considered to be the definitive indication.

During the initial stages of fasting, the body burns stored fat and glucose, which is liberated from stores of glycogen in the muscles and liver. Soon thereafter, the glycogen reserves are metered out more slowly, and protein is converted to glucose. The protein is absorbed from stores in the muscles but also from dead and diseased tissue. My conjecture in this regard is that the remnants of this absorbed tissue are recycled by sending them back to the digestive tract for digestion. That is, normally, digested nutrients in the digestive tract are absorbed into the bloodstream; now, that process is reversed. This conjecture accounts for the fact that, during fasting, the tongue, which is the visible part of the digestive tract, becomes heavily coated, and the extent of this coating decreases as the fast progresses and usually disappears completely when the fast naturally ends and hunger returns. In some cases, where reserves are insufficient to clear out all proteinaceous debris, hunger returns before the tongue clears. That is when fasting must be ended.

Even though the muscle cells release protein, the number of muscle cells is not reduced, which means that after the fast ends and protein is introduced into the diet, the muscle tissue can return to normal. However, some of the fat lacing and surrounding the muscles may not return.

Dangers of Fasting

Fasting is not without danger—those undertaking long fasts on their own are sometimes unable to distinguish fasting from starvation. Disastrous consequences—even death— may ensue. Because a fasting person's sensitivity to physical and emotional stimuli increases dramatically, susceptibility to these factors must be kept in mind. Moreover, it is sometimes necessary to deal with "crises," which can arise as deep-seated poisons leave the body during a long fast. Moreover, breaking the fast properly is of crucial importance. Therefore, it is imperative that anyone considering fasting for even one day become knowledgeable about the subject. *It cannot be overemphasized that any fast longer than three days must be supervised by a competent professional.*

Because breaking a fast correctly is so important, it will be discussed later in this chapter.

How Much Water?

Some people feel that it is necessary to drink a gallon of water every day while fasting. How can an arbitrary amount of water suit a body under constantly changing internal and external conditions? The needs of the body vary tremendously from hour to hour and day to day. On some days, little water is appropriate. On other days more water is required. But most experts agree that a gallon of water is far in excess of any needs. A one-size-fits-all mentality is antithetical to the sensitivity required to fine-tune the intake of water.

On one hand, too much water dilutes toxins and, therefore, reduces the ability of the body to eliminate them. The body then must eliminate this excess water using energy that could otherwise be spent on removing toxins. On the other hand, too little water results in toxins becoming so concentrated that they are difficult to transport out of the body, and these toxins are damaging to the kidneys and other parts of the body. Too little water is much worse than too much, but both extremes are undesirable. Thus, one must strive for the correct amount of water and know the signs of too little or too much.

The criterion that many experts suggest is to drink water based on thirst. Unfortunately, many people have lost their ability to experience thirst reliably because of years of disregarding it and/or drinking carbonated, sugary, caffeinated, or alcoholic beverages instead of pure water. Moreover, during fasting, the tongue is heavily coated and there is a very unpleasant taste in the mouth. Therefore, an awareness of thirst can be masked by these factors. In my experience, it is of value to be aware of changes in bodily energy. When I feel slightly more tired than at other times, I try sipping water. Once the water is going down my throat, the needs of the body will more likely dictate my drinking the correct amount. Observing the color of urine can be misleading. The urine can be very pale yet heavily laden with toxins. However, if the color is darker than that of light beer, I take it as a sign that I am not consuming enough water. Another sign of insufficient water is a muddling of the unusually clear state of mind during fasting.

Again, it is much better to drink too much water rather than too little, so if there is any doubt, err on the side of caution.

Some people believe that drinking their own urine while fasting is advantageous. When water is unavailable and one might die from dehydration, such a measure might be appropriate. Also, there are some forms of therapy whose success stems from drinking one's own *non-fasting* urine. However, during fasting, the urine consists of concentrated toxins that the body can only eliminate through that route. To return these poisons to the bloodstream sabotages the efforts of the body to eliminate them. The idea that it is important to ingest essential nutrients that are in the urine is fallacious because the beneficial effects of fasting rely on depriving the body of nutrients. Moreover, there are no recorded cases of nutritional deficiencies arising from fasting. If anything, the nutrients liberated from diseased and healthy tissues are more than sufficient to prevent a deficiency.

How to Proceed

A fast cannot mitigate the effects of years of wrong eating. Unless bad habits are well on their way to being reversed, they will likely be resumed as soon as the fast ends. Thus, it is important to regard fasting as a tool within a context of many other methods of self-improvement. Before considering fasting, an individual should first make every attempt to become educated about proper diet and apply that knowledge for a period of time. Then, after thus improving the body and preparing it by eating only fruit the day before, a one-day fast can be attempted. After successfully fasting for one day and eating judiciously for a week or so, it is permissible to try another one-day fast. After completing a number of one-day fasts, 36-hour or two-day fasts can be attempted. Eventually, a three-day fast can be tried. Again, *any fast longer than three days must be supervised by an expert.*

Hunger During a Fast

During the first several days of a fast, hunger may be intense. After that, it usually leaves but returns when the body has cleaned itself out or depletes its reserves. Of course, many of us often erroneously think that we are experiencing hunger, which is a physiological need of the body for nutrients. Instead, what we may be experiencing is false hunger due to any number of the following: low blood sugar; an irritation of the lining of the stomach; food-addictions; the discomfort of the body in utilizing reserves; a desire for stimulation; a genuine need for essential nutrients, expressed by a craving for foods of low nutritive value; tiredness experienced as a need for food, thinking about, stimulation from seeing, or smelling food; habituation to regularity; or a desire for distraction from a distasteful task or chore. False hunger may appear during a fast for any of the above reasons and especially when one is exposed to the sight or odor of food, but true hunger is absent.

I have long wondered why hunger leaves during a fast, always to return when fasting is completed or broken early on. I now feel that the following conjecture is correct:

Modern humans eat haphazard combinations of food in amounts impossible to properly digest. The partly digested proteins and putrefactive byproducts find their way into our bloodstream and cells and compromise our immune systems. We get improper amounts of sunlight, and our air and water are polluted with myriad poisons. Our foods are forced to grow on soil that is depleted of essential nutrients and are then devitalized and laced with preservatives, artificial colors, and artificial flavors. Thus, over the years, every cell in our bodies has collected toxins from these factors. During fasting, when we start drawing on our reserves in the order of the least needed first, these toxins are released into the bloodstream at a high rate and must be metabolized by the liver and eliminated by the kidneys. The result of such a burden is nausea and the loss of any interest in food.

The difference between humans of today and those of just 25-thousand years ago is that they were living in touch with nature. They were eating foods in their natural environment, getting optimal amounts of fresh air, sunlight, pure water, and physical activity. When our ancestors of that time were deprived of food for any length of time, their bodies started drawing on their reserves in the order of the least needed first. Because of a healthier lifestyle, their cells would have had substantially less toxic material released into their bloodstream, and they would have been constantly hungry.

Thus, the lack of hunger during fasting appears to result from toxicity, and once all the toxic debris is cleared out, the coating on the tongue leaves and hunger returns. Of course, for someone who is highly toxic and whose vital reserves are depleted before all the toxic debris is cleared out, hunger nevertheless returns as a life-saving expedient. That is why the return of hunger is considered as the definitive sign that a fast must be ended.

Weight-Loss During a Fast

At the beginning of a fast, several pounds of weight per day can be lost. This loss is mostly the contents of the gut and stores of water required to bind excess salt in the tissues. As the excess salt is excreted, weight-loss tapers off to about a pound or less per day. Fig. 11-38 is a graph of typical weight-loss during a lengthy fast.

A Complete Fast

A complete fast is one that is continued to the point of true hunger. The reason for fasting to completion is that, as starvation approaches and the body becomes more desperate for nutriment, it reaches deeper into tissues to retrieve abnormal and morbid tissue. Herbert Shelton, who supervised approximately 40,000 fasts at his health school at San Antonio Texas, reports that, in the case of serious disease, the last several days of a fast can mean the difference between success and failure.

One difficulty experienced during a complete fast is that of well-meaning friends and loved ones who entreat you to break such a fast prematurely. This negative influence can be debilitating and even break a faster's resolve. That is also why it is important to have such a fast supervised by an experienced practitioner, who can be relied upon to guide and reassure you.

Difficulties During a Fast

The first several days of fasting are the most difficult. A powerful appetite for food looms in the forefront. Hunger soon leaves, and unless one actively thinks about food, hunger is not an issue. Tiredness and headaches are common. Sugar-eaters are most prone to the tiredness and headaches resulting from low blood sugar, and coffee drinkers get headaches as they withdraw from their addiction. In fact, many headache remedies contain caffeine, which apparently is an antidote to caffeine withdrawal symptoms. Nausea and even vomiting can occur. The coating on one's tongue is very distasteful and the feeling in the mouth has been likened to "the inside of a motorman's glove." As the gaseous toxins released into the bloodstream are expelled via the lungs, the breath becomes foul, but as the fast nears completion, the breath becomes very sweet. One experiences periods of elation, well-being, and surprising spurts of energy, and there are periods of weakness and giddiness. Highly spiritual experiences are not uncommon.

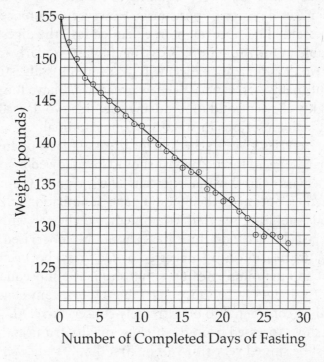

Fig. 11-38. *A graph of the weight loss during a recent 28-day fast done by the author. Please note that the vertical axis is broken and does not start at zero. The fast was begun in August, 2006. The graph plots weight on the morning of each day of the fast versus the number of complete days fasted. Note how the daily amount of weight lost decreases during the first week but then levels off to approximately 3/4 pound per day as the fast progresses.*

Breaking a Fast

The hardest part of fasting is breaking it properly. Here is where strong resolve is necessary not to succumb to the ravenous appetite that develops and jump back to prior habits of wrong eating.

Arnold De Vries[85] and others tell of disastrous medical results of improperly breaking long fasts. For a healthy person, breaking a short fast is less critical. However, carefully breaking any fast extends and greatly augments its beneficial health and educational effects.

There are many ways of breaking a fast. Those who supervise fasts use freshly squeezed (not bottled!) juices, and others use fresh fruit eaten slowly. Bragg[86] uses cooked tomatoes. His next meal consists of a raw salad of carrots and grated cabbage, with the juice of an orange squeezed over it. The Chinese use congee, which is rice that is boiled in a large amount of water for a long time until it breaks down into a soup-like porridge. Congee is said to be very soothing to the digestive tract and conducive to a natural return of peristalsis. However, adherence to time-tested rules is essential because, after an extended fast, the digestive organs are unable to fully function. Breaking the fast properly (absolute minimum of two days on a juice diet) will result in one's digestive tract functioning optimally—an experience few ever have. I have found that eating thoroughly chewed solid food during the first two days after breaking a fast is not a serious mistake but is not optimal.

On page 66, De Vries gives a schedule for breaking fasts of any length. He suggests that a one-to three-day fast should be followed by one full day during which a glass of freshly made juice is slowly sipped at 2-hour intervals. This procedure optimizes the digestion and assimilation of the juice. Afterward, foods should be selected, combined, and chewed with utmost care. Whereas fasts longer than three days should be supervised, for reference purposes, the relationship (suggested by De Vries) between the length of a fast and the number of days that should be subsequently spent on a juice diet for longer fasts is given in Table 11-2. By any standard, this regimen would be considered to be extremely conservative. All juices must be raw and freshly expressed from the highest quality fruits and vegetables. They must be sipped very slowly. The first day, the juice should be diluted in half with water. Carrot juice is considered the best one because of its balance of nutrients.

---

85. Arnold De Vries, *Therapeutic Fasting*, pp. 63–64.
86. Paul C. Bragg, *The Miracle of Fasting*, p. 75.

Table 11-2. The relationship between the length of a fast and the suggested number of subsequent days to be spent on a juice diet.

Length of Fast (days)	Length of Juice Diet (days)
1–3	1
4–8	2
9–15	3
16–24	4
25–35	5
over 35	6

A more realistic, time-tested regimen for breaking a fast is given by Shelton[87] for a fast longer than 20 days (Table 11-3). Shelton permits no between-meal or after-supper eating and emphasizes going slowly!

The Difference Between Fasting and Anorexia

Fasting is total abstinence from food for a relatively short period of time determined by natural conditions. The motivation for fasting is not weight-loss but improved health. Fasting involves an application of millennia-old principles to attain better health (or in some cases a heightened mental and spiritual state). During fasting, hunger is naturally absent and returns when the fast ends. The results of fasting are all positive: improved health and longevity and removal of toxic and morbid matter from the body. Energy and outlook are improved.

Table 11-3. A regimen used by Shelton for breaking a fast longer than 20 days. Note that, during each of the first two days, the same total amount of juice is taken but in different ways.

Day 1	1/2 glass of juice every hour (not after 8 PM)
Day 2	whole glass of juice every 2 hours (not after 8 PM)
Day 3	Breakfast: one orange
	Lunch: two oranges
	Supper: three oranges
Day 4	Breakfast: citrus or other fruits
	Lunch: vegetable salad (no salt or dressing), one cooked green vegetable
	Supper: fruit
Day 5	Breakfast: fruit
	Lunch: salad, two cooked vegetables and baked potato or small quantity of protein
	Supper: fruit and yogurt (if desired)
Day 6	Same as day 5
Day 7	Eat normal amounts of regular food

87. Herbert M. Shelton, *Fasting Can Save Your Life*, Natural Hygiene Press, Inc., Chicago, IL, 1964, pp. 71–72

Anorexia seems to stem not from the desire to be healthy but to be very thin, an erroneous idea promulgated by the movie and fashion industries. In anorexia, an insufficient amount of food is eaten over an extended period, causing a lack of protein, vitamins, minerals, essential fatty acids, and other essential nutrients. There is a state of mind that hypnotically blots out hunger, which results in malnutrition (a state that has never been recorded to occur during fasting). Anorexia ends from outside pressure, forced feeding, or death from malnutrition.

Why is Fasting Disregarded?

When I became interested in fasting in the late 1960s, I wanted to read every book on the subject. The books I was able to find were available only in health-food stores with large book sections. When I had exhausted these sources, it dawned on me to look in the medical library at New York University, where I taught physics. There were only two books on fasting in the card catalog. One of these books was lost, and the other was written in the early 1900s. The available book was a study of only one individual. The authors did not seem to know much about any aspect of fasting, which they referred to as *starvation*. Their conclusions were that the subject of the study, a man in good health, lost a substantial amount of fat and muscle mass and was not as strong at the end as he was at the beginning. Other than that, the book did not seem to discuss much else or say anything negative or positive.

I wondered how such an inexpensive, non-invasive, and effective healing tool about which so many books have been written could be so completely disregarded by a profession dedicated to bringing sick people back to health. Even today, many "alternative" physicians seem not to consider that fasting could ever have any value.

Over the years, I have formulated an explanation for what I consider to be the medical profession's disregard of fasting and other time-honored areas of knowledge. The reader is encouraged to do likewise.

12

Self-Development

"Every moment is an opportunity for enlightenment."

WHAT IS SELF-DEVELOPMENT?

M any people who study any discipline—including Taiji—are mainly interested in attaining benefits such as physical and mental skills, personal power, martial skills, physical health, increased financial assets, or others' respect. Such attainments develop the ego, or "lower self." *Self-development* here refers to the *self* that is beyond the physical—beyond designations of female/male, young/old, rich/poor, educated/uneducated, etc. This latter self can be called our *higher self* and is really the one that we are here to develop.

When we talk about ego in a spiritual or martial-arts context, we are referring to the part of our identity that is formed by the outside world. Such an identity is in contrast to our identity as a consciousness whose implicitly understood goal is to learn and grow in accordance with our true purpose for being in a human body. Our egos are formed from (often false) ideas that come from our parents, schooling, friends, newspapers, television, movies, entertainment, and religion. Moreover, our bodies have preprogrammed responses driven by emotions, sexual drives, and a need to eat and sleep. Our lower selves, or egos, therefore, express biological needs, raw emotions, and false development. Our lower selves begin at birth and end with death. On the other hand, our higher selves are indestructible and have neither a beginning nor an end.

To the extent that we see the effects of our raw emotions, biological needs, and false, outside influences and put them in their proper perspective through meditation and studying spiritual teachings, we are on the road to the kind of development that most people inwardly seek but from which they have been sidetracked.

The basic goal is to see things as they are. The first step is recognizing the degree to which we are limited by our emotions, biological needs, and having taken on others' ideas. Taiji has Buddhist underpinnings but is not primarily a self-development teaching in the above sense. It is possible to progress in Taiji and miss opportunities for self-development because that aspect has not been systematized and specifically taught. On the other hand, once you have been exposed to Buddhist and other teachings, myriad opportunities for self-development abound in doing Taiji form and push-hands.

The following are some of the self-development concepts that I have been taught. Where appropriate, the aspect of Taiji form and push-hands practice will be linked to the self-development concepts discussed.

To know the truth of the above and following claims, which parallel those of Buddhism, one needs to look beyond one's upbringing, schooling, and religion. Accepting these claims is not done on the basis of faith but on experiencing their truth, mutual consistency, and utility emerging over time.

BASIC CONCEPTS OF SELF-DEVELOPMENT

Everything is for Learning

Injuries, emotional traumas, personal losses, setbacks in relationships, frustrations, harsh criticism, and even disease are all for learning and self-development. The following phrase sums up this truth succinctly:

"Every misfortune has within it the seeds of an even greater benefit."

When we are in physical or emotional pain, it is very difficult to see things in perspective. But, at that moment, seeing things objectively is crucial, for that is when a major opportunity for growth appears. At such a time, negative emotions are at their peak and prevent objectivity. Here is where extending the principles of Taiji can be of much help in minimizing the effect of negative emotions. First, it is important to understand the role of emotions.

Emotions

Emotions can be finely tuned, valuable tools, ready at all times to alert us to all manner of important situations, or they can take us over and turn our lives and those around us into a nightmare. Unfortunately, we tend to allow our emotions to overstep their usefulness, control us, and separate us from our higher mental and spiritual aspects. Television and movies exploit negative emotions, which further increase our susceptibility to them. Therefore, an understanding of the nature and role of emotions is essential to spiritual growth.

Our emotions are the remnants of the instinctual preprogramming of the lower animals from which we have descended. Lower animals lack sufficient mental and spiritual development and, therefore, require instincts (preprogrammed responses) to enable them to survive. Fear, for example, is required so that an animal knows when it is in danger. Moreover, anger evokes fear in other animals and causes them to recognize that they may be in danger if they harm the angry individual. Thus, fear and anger are protective because they allow effective reaction, albeit on a low level. The protective nature of such emotions has evolved to ensure the survival of the species—not necessarily the individual and his/her development. To develop spiritually, we humans must go beyond the purely preprogrammed, instinctual level and evolve toward directing the movement of the material world in concord with cosmic principles rather than being directed by them.

Instincts are a "heavy-handed" way of interacting with the environment because they do not involve any higher thought, which would be required for any delicate handling of a situation. Emotions are devoid of higher reason. Emotions are highly affected by such things as the weather, the phases of the moon, and items in the diet such as coffee, chocolate, sugar, alcohol, artificial sweeteners, and animal flesh. Moreover, emotions are frequently contradictory and are destructive to us, to others, and our spiritual growth.

Consider the following emotions, which have negative effects when they overstep their bounds: fear, anger, remorse, regret, guilt, pity, self-pity, hate, jealousy, envy, impatience, and sorrow. The over-expression and over-cultivation of such emotions are at the expense of spiritual growth. Even the more positive emotions, some of which are love, sympathy, and empathy, are activated by the media more as a form of entertainment than in any spiritually uplifting manner.

If we are to go beyond responding to the world in a preprogrammed manner, we must understand and go beyond our emotions. First, we must become expert at feeling and expressing emotions. The next stage is to transcend (not suppress) emotions by using our creative intelligence to deal with situations in an uplifting manner. As the creative process manifests itself in its unlimited range of action, the emotions begin to take a less-active role because they are required less. Why should a person experience an emotion, such as fear, when that person is fully utilizing a creative ability far more effective in dealing with whatever situation is at hand? Of course, such strong built-in responses do not fall away that quickly, and it takes a substantial amount of work in using the creative part of our mind before a change for the better is noticeable.

Instead of ignoring, submerging, or suppressing our emotions, we must transcend their overwhelming influence so that our thoughts and actions are harmonious with our spirit. Then, the usefulness of emotions increases as the control they have over us fades into the background.

Releasing

One of the most basic principles in Taiji is to release all unnecessary muscular action (song). In addition to its value in improving physical health, song is the physical precursor to releasing our attachments to unneeded emotions, ideas, possessions, jobs, and interpersonal relationships.

There is much evidence that memories of physical and emotional traumas are embedded in the musculature of our bodies. By maintaining corresponding muscular tensions, we tend to protect ourselves from having these memories percolate into our awareness. Because these tensions are protective, we have a strong attachment to them and feel unprotected when they are released. We become so used to these tensions that they seem to represent our very identity. Thus, we have difficulty in releasing these tensions.

When doing Taiji or Qigong movements, we gradually release unneeded physical tension and open the body. By doing so, we are, in a way, allowing the memories of these traumas to rise closer to the surface. To the extent that we are successful in releasing our habitual muscular patterns through practicing song, we are beginning the process of releasing the corresponding emotional traumas. Moreover, and possibly more importantly, we are practicing releasing not only our tensions but *any* unneeded attachment. By recognizing that song has effects beyond the physical, we can more efficiently utilize its self-developmental aspects. The following story illustrates the benefits of releasing when it is time to do so:

In 1975, I got a job at a public high school. Early in my second year there, I became quite dissatisfied with the teaching load and the recurring friction between the administration and faculty. I started to feel that I should not return after finishing out the academic year, but I felt very insecure about doing so because, right then, the job market was very poor.

One night, I had a very vivid dream: I had just entered a room and was holding open the door through which I had just entered. There was a closed door at the other end of the room. I knew that if the door I was holding were to close, it would lock behind me, and the door at the other end of the room might also be locked; in short, I might be trapped in that room! I decided to take a chance and let the door close. When I got to the other door, I found it unlocked. I opened it and was now in another room with another door at the other end. The same sequence of letting one door close and finding the next door unlocked was repeated twice more.

When I awoke, I knew exactly what this dream meant. It had addressed my fear of what might happen should I resign my present job. The fear was that quitting this job during a poor job market might result in another job not materializing. The dream had reassured me that if I "closed the door" of my present teaching job, the door to my next job would open.

Soon thereafter, I told my chairman that I would not be back next year. He was amazed that I had made such a decision so early in the year, during a very bad lull in the job market and without another position lined up. He advised me to reconsider, saying, "The economy is very bad right now. Others would give their right arm to have your job." Nevertheless, I was resolved to quit at the end of the school year.

Over a year went by without my securing another full-time job. I taught Taiji classes at Sarah Lawrence College, my own Taiji classes, and physics at New York University during the summer. After the summer was over, the chairman of the New York University physics department telephoned me. He told me that a very "upscale" private high school was looking for a substitute physics teacher. I accepted without any thought other than it might be fun. After a few days of subbing, I was asked to stay the year. I remained there for twenty-seven years until I retired!

Had I not released the previous job, I would not have been available to do the substitute teaching, which led to a permanent position that was right for me.

Direct Versus Indirect Experiencing

One of the most important distinctions that can be made for those aspiring to spiritual growth is that between direct and indirect experiencing. Most of our experiencing is indirect; that is, it comes into our awareness through our physical senses of sight, hearing, smell, etc., and is then processed by using language and a conceptual framework influenced by others. Examples of such outside influences include that from our parents, schooling, friends, and the various media (TV, movies, newspapers, etc.). Much of what comes into our ears and eyes is filled with distortion—some of it unintended but much of it with an agenda. Consider that the food and medical industries each take in approximately one trillion dollars per year. They and other such industries have a strong motivation to maintain or increase their profits by molding the public's conceptual framework. For example, if people did not think that "breakfast is the most important meal of the day," the breakfast-cereal industries would lose a substantial income. Example after example of a similar nature can be cited. Much of what we believe and even the nature of how we experience things such as entertainment, food, art, and music are highly colored by our indirect experiencing.

In contrast, what we experience directly from our bodies and from what we see and hear in our mind's eyes and ears is very different. Direct experiencing occurs to the greatest degree during meditation. Of course sitting meditation is the most common example, but doing Taiji form and push-hands, Yoga, walking, and many other activities can also be akin to sitting meditation although not as intense. In meditation, there are no emotions, no positive or negative characterizations through language, and no thought of "self"—just direct experiencing. During sitting meditation, nothing comes in through any of our physical senses, only through the mind. During Taiji, Yoga, or walking, some of the physical senses are active, but there can be much direct experiencing.

Through direct experiencing, whether partial (as in Taiji) or complete (as in sitting meditation), we experience a "truth" that is undefiled by the mass thinking, with its distortions, prejudices, and agendas; the profit motives of industry; or our own emotions, with their preprogrammed and compelling nature, all of which are very limiting to our spiritual growth.

If we are to see things as they are rather than through others' eyes, we must put into perspective that which is distorted and laden with an agenda other than that pertaining to our growth. Ultimate stability and creative usage of mind cannot ever be developed when outside influences color our thinking.

Opening and Closing the Front of the Body

For various reasons, we tend to close the front of the body much more than we should. One reason is that, in today's world, many of us spend much time sitting at desks, where we read, write, and work on computers. Another reason that we close the front is that it helps us feel more protected in dealing with others who are competitive, aggressive, and confrontational. It should be noted that the opening of the front of the body referred to here is not that required of military cadets, which involves pulling the shoulders back by contracting muscles in the back. Instead, it is allowing the front of the body to expand naturally, as it does when allowed to do so.

All Taiji movements open and close the front, but movements such as "Single Whip," "White Crane Spreads Wings," "Repulse Monkey," "Diagonal Flying," and "Parting the Wild Horse's Mane" do so to a greater extent. "White Crane Spreads Wings" and "Fair Lady Works Shuttles" open the front of the body in two directions, horizontally and vertically. Some movements close the front, which is then opened by the next movement and then again closed by the movement after. An example of such an alternation is "Needle at Sea Bottom," "Fan Through the Back," and "Turn and Chop with Fist."

During Taiji practice, it is of value to allow the entire front of the body to subtly respond to the opening and closing of the arms and legs rather than have the movement come solely from the large joints. It will be discovered that doing so noticeably increases the flow of qi throughout the body.

In cultivating opening the front of your body, it is useful to imagine yourself lying on your back on a sandy beach during summer, feeling the warmth of the sun on the front of your body. Imagine the clouds in the sky, a cool breeze, and the sounds of surf and seagulls. Then recreate the deep state of relaxation of the front of the body that would accompany this situation. If necessary, this image can be employed while lying on your back on the floor.

Opening the front of the body is more than a physical action—it has several self-developmental aspects. One aspect is that practicing opening the front brings out responses that are honest and "from the heart." Others feel safer and less likely to become confrontational, and should a confrontation happen, it is more quickly dissipated.

Even more importantly, being practiced in opening the body helps you not only to be honest with others but also with yourself, both of which are closely related. Self-honesty is a necessary condition to spiritual growth. The self-honesty acquired is not a brutal one that punishes but a soft, understanding, rewarding one.

LAUGHTER

Laughter opens the body in a natural and highly beneficial manner. Laughter is a very basic almost "soul-to-soul" mode of communication between people. It is, of course, a mistake to contrive laughter, but when humorous situations arise, say in Taiji class, that is when qi flows most freely and everyone feels interconnected in a highly beneficial manner. The following is my attempt to analyze what humor is:

There are a number of interactions in our daily lives so commonplace that viewing them objectively is very difficult. Laughter is one of these. A visitor from another world observing people engaged in laughter might at first think that they were experiencing excruciating pain. When people laugh, they grimace, emit sharp cries, wipe away real or imaginary tears, and might even double up as if in excruciating pain. The visitor might easily conclude that there is a relationship between anguish and laughter and might be surprised to learn that communication evoking laughter is eagerly sought.

Close scrutiny reveals that humor always involves a veiled reference to sorrow. The success of humor depends on the fact that *the understanding of one another's sorrow is more strongly conveyed than the sorrow to which it refers.* The fact that another understands our sorrow is very uplifting to us, but this understanding must be communicated through a clever and indirect means; otherwise, the reference to pain will predominate, and the attempt at humor will fail.

The success of the humor is acknowledged by simultaneously expressing the emotions of joy and sorrow. The joy is experienced because we know that another understands our pain. The cries and gestures of anguish express the depth of pain referred to.

Ticklishness, an interesting phenomenon ending in laughter, can be similarly interpreted. Tickling involves lightly touching a vulnerable and sensitive spot such as the ribs. The person doing the tickling communicates that he understands the other's vulnerability in that region by applying just the right pressure below the threshold of pain.

The pun is a type of humor that alludes to the high degree of frustration it is possible to experience from wrongly interpreting an important communication having two different meanings.

In slapstick humor, we laugh, not because we enjoy seeing another be hurt but because it expresses an understanding of what it feels like to be hurt.

There is a fine line between (a) reverence for life and the laws of nature and (b) a disruption of these laws. It may be that even sadism has its roots in a desire to see the forces of nature come into play under adversity and that the sadist is displaying a perverted appreciation for harmony. In this light, sadism can be thought of as an extreme and perverted version of what sports, literature, drama, art, and music accomplish in a less harmful and often more-socially uplifting manner.

NEGATIVITY

Negativity is a mental attitude wherein we view the events of our lives to be under the control and direction of others. This mental attitude is accompanied by the sense that we are impotent to institute change. Negativity manifests itself as a perversion of our sense of perfection; when we make a mistake—and making mistakes is how we learn—our disappointment in our imperfection is allowed to overshadow our deeper, more subtle knowledge that, in the long run, the situational harm of the mistake is less important than the long-term benefit of learning from that mistake.

Negativity breeds more negativity. The more we think negatively, the more seemingly justified our negative thinking becomes. Entrenchment in negativity divorces us from using our creative faculties for growth and harmony.

We are surrounded by negativity from the media and our interactions with others. How do we neutralize or wash away the negativity that we inevitably accept from the outside world? One way is to commune with nature. We could go to the top of a mountain where there is fresh pure air and where the only sounds are that of insects, birds, trees, grass, wind, and water—not sounds of jet aircraft, diesel trucks, drag racers, high-wattage hi-fi sets in passing cars, box radios, and dogs that bark and yelp for hours; where there are no cigar butts, empty soda and beer cans, graffiti, or negative people; where the odor is of trees, flowers, and plants rather than cigarette smoke, car, truck, and bus exhaust, the effluvia of factories, and the smell of flame-broiled carcasses of animals; and where the only sights are those of clouds, vegetation, and natural animal life.

The big question is, "Where is such a place?" As the world gets more and more over-populated, pristine mountain tops are increasingly remote. However, there is such a place—you! Within each of us is the complete universe, wherein all of the laws of nature operate. We are each a microcosm of the universe. We can temporarily let go of our mechanical everyday thinking by becoming attuned to inward, natural processes such as our breathing or the colors and images that appear before our closed eyes. Or we can listen to inner sounds, which can sometimes exceed in beauty any of the greatest works of music. In this way we can connect with that part of ourselves which is free of the conditioning, opinions, ideas, etc., of others. Taijiquan, meditation, Yoga, music, and even certain ways of dancing are some of the many ways that one can shed the negativity that surrounds us.

A Story. When I was a graduate student in physics at New York University, I had an outstanding professor, James P. Hurley, who was fond of creating physics problems that stemmed from the homework problems. One day he created a problem that he was unable to do. After unsuccessfully working on this problem for days, he happened to notice that the very same problem was among the homework exercises given in the text. Immediately, Hurley knew that the problem was one he could easily do and solved it on the spot. In the next class, Hurley marveled at how the thought that you may not be able to do something prevents you from doing it.

If you think you can do a thing or think you can't do a thing, you're right.

—Henry Ford

Instead of feeling embarrassed, Hurley utilized the situation for self-understanding and selflessly shared it with the class.

REGRET

When we regret our actions in the past, we have lost sight of the fact that everything is for learning. We also are not recognizing and forgiving our limitations of the past. If we could see the total picture objectively, we would realize that everything we did in the past was a result of our development at that time, and now that we have the increased understanding from the experience, we are in a position not to make the same mistake again.

Reviewing past mistakes emotionally is a form of self-punishment. Self-punishment masks the very objectivity leading to the growth necessary for not making the same mistakes again.

The Law of Attraction

The law of attraction states that you get what you need for your growth and that of others.

> *"When the student is ready, the teacher arrives; when the teacher is ready, the student arrives."*

To the extent that you are contributing to the growth of others, say by writing a book that will assist others or by other actions, you will attract whatever will help that information to get out. If you are not growing and not contributing to others' growth, you may get what you need in the form of "shock treatment," as illustrated by the following example:

One of my private Taiji students complained that he had had a succession of accidents, "none of them my fault." When he drove me somewhere, I realized that he was cutting things so close that he was causing accidents even if they were technically not his fault. After another such accident, his insurance company denied him insurance. He had to get new, much more costly insurance and was required to take a driver-safety course. After taking the course, he confided in me that he had learned that he *was* cutting things too close. His bad driving attracted accidents even if they were not technically his fault. Being denied insurance, etc., was "shock treatment" that helped him correct his errors. Had he not changed, he might have been killed or seriously injured, or he might have killed or seriously injured others.

Unfortunately, the wrong way of interacting with our surroundings keeps coming back like weeds in a garden. But there is a difference between weeds cropping up in a neglected garden and those in a garden that is weeded on an ongoing basis. Although there is always more to do, by working on self-development regularly, progress occurs even if it is sometimes masked by new challenges.

RESPONSIBILITY

Responsibility is a mental attitude wherein we accept that our own thinking and consequent actions—not those of others—are of primary importance in our lives. It is a rejection of the goal orientation we all learned in school or from parents or society. It is an awareness that our past actions, however wayward, have value for our growth. Any other emphasis is at best wasteful and, at worst, self-punishment and, therefore, detrimental to true growth.

At a certain point a "life-or-death" decision may have to be made and implemented. That is, we must choose the correct one of two opposite directions. One direction leads toward harmony and self-evolution, whereas the other direction leads toward spiritual sleep. Once this decision is made, it is implemented by a devoted recognition of negativity in all its myriad forms and by reaffirming our commitment to responsibility. Here is where what might be termed *self-denial* comes into play. We must expel negativity, which may be a long-standing habit, using all the power of our being. Over and over again, this cleansing process must be repeated. As time goes on, similar to the manner in which water wears away rocks, the persistence of our expectation will bear a monumental result.

The levels of development are: (0) Total entrenchment in negativity; (1) the life-or-death decision; (2) blameless analysis of past actions to uncover negative thinking and to ask, "What would have been the responsible action?" (3) blameless analysis of situations in progress and an alteration of action for the better in these situations; and (4) natural, correct action involving no negativity.

The importance of a spiritual teacher and of meditation is substantial. A teacher inspires us, reminds us of our evolution, and shows us a more direct path. Meditation frees us of our preprogrammed, mechanized thinking, and brings us more into touch with higher levels of our consciousness and with other consciousnesses.

DEALING WITH PERSONAL POWER

In engaging in any study for self-development, especially a martial art, personal power grows substantially but often imperceptibly. At a certain point, it is important to realize that just as positive thoughts about others can be beneficial to them, negative thoughts can be at least as damaging. As you develop power, you cannot afford the luxury of even having negative thoughts about another person because the effects of such thoughts can be more far-reaching and damaging than you think—not only to that person but to yourself. If you outwardly express anger toward another, that person will have a better chance of having the protection to deal with and learn from it than if you surreptitiously have angry thoughts. When a person of power deals with another negatively and in secret, it is tantamount to practicing black magic.

Of course, the ill effects of such negativity are not limited to that on the other person; they affect you at least as much. Anger (unless expressed as a judiciously designed tactic, devoid of emotion) reinforces our emotional preprogramming rather than helping to uplift us. In short, attainment of power must parallel spiritual development. We see the negative effects, world-wide, of scientific power unleashed on the environment and peoples of the world in the absence of a spiritual basis. Let us not act so in our individual lives.

My meditation teacher, Alice Holtman, used to say, "If you are angry, it is because the other person's actions have found a sensitive spot in you. Instead of nurturing anger, repair the weakness that was uncovered in your understanding. When you act from anger, you are off balance." She also quoted Buddha, who said, "Your enemies are your best friends" because they show you what you need to learn.

SELF-DENIAL

Self-denial is an element often emphasized in spiritual teachings. Some feel that by denying the physical aspect of ourselves along with its corresponding mental attachments, we strengthen our mental and spiritual aspect. This ideology has some merit but falls short of being a direct route to unfoldment. Self-denial is duality. To deny any aspect of ourselves is to have contempt for nature. True, a certain degree of inner strength is attainable by such actions as, for example, relinquishing possessions or withstanding extreme physical pain, and it may even be that these actions are appropriate at a certain stage of spiritual development. However, the direct route involves no such actions. That is not to say that we should coddle ourselves either. Self-mastery is attained through balance and harmony.

The root of all wrong action or disharmony on the physical level is wrong thinking. Rather than denying the material manifestation of the wrong thinking, and hoping that eradicating the manifestation will result in any good, we must give up the wrong thinking itself. How is this transformation accomplished? It may seem that we are doomed to failure, for how can something distorted act upon itself to free itself from distortion? How can wrong thinking become right thinking?

First, we are not going it alone. We are surrounded by other intelligence, which is available to help us to an unlimited degree. Second, it is important to realize that each of us has a "higher self," which is free of distorted thinking. The higher self is not merely an abstraction. Rather, it is something to which we have access and which we almost must use force to disregard. Here is where meditation plays a key role. In meditation we subdue the mechanized, opinionated, preprogrammed thinking of our everyday life and nurture a type of thought involving our eternal wisdom. In the meditative state, our thoughts cease to be in terms of language (which involves the distortions and limitations of human thought and expression in general), and they link directly with our highest wisdom.

A strong start in the right direction is accepting that we are not going it alone and that we possess a higher knowledge that can be brought to bear. Such an acceptance means that we are moving out of negativity towards responsibility.

CRITICISM

The help we get with our growth takes many forms. A very important form is criticism from others. It is better to get criticism—even if hurtful—than to suffer physical injury or sickness, both of which stem from uncorrected, wayward thinking. Even criticism that is misguided, unfounded and malicious still has value in prompting us to re-evaluate our ideas and strengthen us.

Criticism can also take the form of "accidents," injuries, ill health, broken relationships, etc.

TALKING

The spoken word has tremendous power. It is difficult to imagine what life would be like without speech. Words have the ability to communicate highly abstract thoughts with great efficiency. These days, there are numerous ways that speech can be almost instantaneously transmitted over large distances or stored and later played back.

Under some circumstances, though, speech has several negative aspects not commonly recognized. One such aspect is that words, by their very nature, limit our thinking.

Words embody concepts that are common to a large number of people; otherwise, words would not have a communicative aspect. When ideas are expressed using words, those unique and highly individual thoughts, for which words are inadequate, become inhibited. That is, we implicitly know the limitations of verbal expression and thus automatically tend to disregard certain delicate and unique thoughts because words cannot express them. This danger holds for people with a strong command of language as well as those with a limited command. The more we attempt to express thoughts using language, the better we get at minimizing those thoughts that are unique to us and inexpressible in words. This limitation not only applies to communication but, more importantly, to our thought processes.

Next, the words we use have embedded in them the distortions, misconceptions, biases, emotions, prejudices, etc., of others. When we use these words, we subtly accept to a certain degree the premises of the underlying distortions, misconceptions, biases, and emotions, prejudices, etc. This concept is becoming increasingly recognized and being addressed by eliminating expressions that marginalize certain segments of the population. For example, *chairman* conveys a subliminal message that only men act in managerial capacities, whereas *chairperson*, does not.

By verbally expressing certain thoughts, we expose ourselves to another's response, which can be negative and harmful. Not that we must altogether avoid expressing our thoughts, many of which help us and others to learn and grow and which elicit valuable responses. Rather, we should be aware of the risk in certain situations for which another's negativity can harmfully sway us over the threshold. Exercising verbal restraint is especially important for students beginning a discipline requiring much dedication, patience, and ability to withstand discouragement. Beginners are enthusiastic but have a shaky foothold. Because of this susceptibility, beginners should be wary of discussing or exhibiting what they have learned to others; another's scorn for something not understood can easily discourage them to the point of not continuing.

Whenever embarking on some new task, either at odds with establishment thinking (such as a self-healing program) or involving difficulty and discouragement (such as a weight-loss diet), it is important to be very mindful to be reserved about expressing this resolve. While many will be supportive, others, without realizing their impact, might say negative things.

Even if we are prepared for such negativity, it nevertheless has a subliminal effect on our resolve. Or, if we are not treading a beaten path, it amplifies any vestige of self-doubt we may have. Alice Holtman often said, "If you have a spiritual question, don't ask others' opinions. Rather, go into meditation. Any question you have will be resolved in three days *at the very most.*"

Finally, we must observe the implications of the words that we think and say, and seek to eliminate those that have a negative or limiting effect. Whenever we have a thought or say something, it has the capacity to program our subconscious mind. In the words of Alice Holtman, "The subconscious mind is like a slave. It will do whatever you tell it. That is how hypnosis works. We must not tell our subconscious anything that will sabotage our progress." For example, if a student keeps saying, "I know that I am going to fail this test," it can actually sabotage success. Even if the student does not believe it, his or her subconscious will.

It is crucial that the limitations and pitfalls of language not only be understood but be counterbalanced through meditation, during which experiencing occurs directly, without the use of language.

INTUITION

My meditation teacher, Alice Holtman, used to say that intuition is the totality of our experience and knowledge being brought to bear. Of course, we have knowledge and experience of which we are not aware. Some of it comes from past lives, and some of it comes from information from outside intelligence percolating through to our awareness. The following is an interesting account of how intuition sometimes works:

One of my Taiji classmates (Ms. Y) had a loft in New York City's Chinatown, which she let a group of us use for Taiji push-hands practice. One day, as we all left the building, Ms. Y noticed spray-painted markings on the sidewalk. She exclaimed to all of us that these marks meant that something terrible was going to happen to the building in which she had her loft. All of us laughingly reassured her that these innocuous marks, along with thousands of others throughout the city, were put there by Con Edison to mark electric lines buried below. A few days later, the entire building was set on fire and burnt down. Ms. Y was lucky to escape alive.

Here is a case of intuition, rationalized in terms of irrelevant happenings but, nevertheless, correct perceptions.

DREAMS

Dreams are an extremely valuable resource for self-development. In the words of Alice Holtman, "A dream not analyzed is like a letter unopened." Whereas psychologists have studied dreams for about a century, occult teachings such as yoga have extensively studied dreams for millennia. In fact dreams have dimensions beyond those included in established psychiatric practice. Aside from those dreams that reflect psychological states of the person dreaming, dreams frequently have an aspect that goes beyond the consciousness of the dreamer. Some dreams are prophetic. Others are warnings. Still others contain severe distortions and are almost incapable of dependable analysis. The limitation of modern science in studying dreams (and, for that matter, other psychological phenomena) stems from its unwillingness to accept the possibility that knowledge and thoughts of another consciousness can be transmitted directly without any conventionally understood physical mechanism.

Once the possibility that dreams may contain knowledge beyond that possessed by the person dreaming is incorporated in dream analysis, many dreams that are totally perplexing and apparently meaningless become both transparent and valuable. The greatest difficulty is that dreams containing information from without are frequently symbolic and present interpretive challenges.

If we do not accept the existence of planes other than the physical one, we mistake dreams for occurrences on the physical plane, and they are not. When people who associate reality totally with the physical plane have experiences on any other plane, they automatically assume that what is happening must be on the physical plane. This distortion shapes the whole experience of dreams. When we awaken from a dream, we may think that the experience of the dream did not "really" happen and brush it off. However, the experience *was* real; it just was a reality of a different dimension of existence.

When one becomes more aware of or accepting of reality beyond physical reality, then dreams increasingly take on a different tone. If while dreaming, you have an awareness that what you are experiencing is not taking place on the physical plane, that eliminates a basic distortion, and you are much more able to utilize the experience constructively.

Here are a few of my dreams and my interpretations of them. The interpretations are just that: interpretations. They are certainly not offered as proof of anything. In fact, I would be disappointed should the reader blindly accept my interpretations of these dreams—or of anything else for that matter. Instead, the following are offered to expose the reader to a conceptual framework that is typical of those who study meditation, healing, and various Yogic teachings and their Western offshoots.

Dream 1 (several interconnected dreams)

When I was in my late teens, a life-long friend, Michael, committed suicide. He had always acted strangely, and his behavior had become so extreme that all of his friends—including me—shunned him. Eventually, he was institutionalized and became the subject of institutional experimentation with drugs for psychosis.

Soon after Michael's suicide, I met him in a dream. In the dream I was surprised and said to him, "Michael! I thought you were dead!" To this he replied, "That's what everyone says. Can't you see that I am alive?"

This dream recurred in slightly different forms a number of times over the next few years. Each time I saw Michael I again believed him and would say to myself, "I guess I was wrong." Upon awakening, I would realize that I had been fooled. Each time, the dream vividly pervaded my waking thoughts afterward.

Years later, after studying occult teachings, I reluctantly began to entertain the possibility of the consciousness continuing after death. Some of the books I read asserted that people who strongly reject the idea that their consciousness may continue after death frequently do not accept that they are dead when they actually are. They can continue to believe for years that they are alive. Using their minds, they create in the astral world an illusion of earthly phenomena, including the most minute detail. Of course, this state would be considered a severe distortion on their part, which impedes their growth.

Just as it is important for living beings in the physical plane to know the meaning of life, it is equally important for astral dwellers, who have left their physical bodies, to know the meaning of their existence on that plane.

My realization that Michael had the problem of not accepting his death influenced future dreams involving him. In the next dream, I met him at a party. I was immediately aware that what was happening was not in the physical plane. I said to him, "How are things?" He replied, "Better." I said, "Do you realize yet that you are dead?" This question seemed to shock him so much that I thought about it, and, in the dream, it dawned on me that perhaps he had, by now, been reborn into a new body and was not "dead." I rephrased the question: "Do you realize that you committed suicide eighteen years ago?" (My arithmetic in the dream state was quite accurate.) He looked relieved and replied, "Yes." I asked, "How did you find out?" He replied, "My mother told me." I snapped back, "I tried to tell you for *years*, and you didn't believe me." The dream ended. I felt that he had improved quite a bit, and that perhaps he *was* now in a new body.

In my next and last dream with Michael, he showed me a manuscript and said, "Would you like to hear some music that I have written?" Although I dreaded hearing it, I said, "Yes." He sat down at a piano and started to play the most incredibly beautiful music. His hands flew deftly over the keyboard, and from the music and the way he moved his hands, I knew that he had completely recovered from the distress that prompted him to take his own life. I then noticed his father sitting by his side, beaming with joy and pride. This was the first time his father was in a dream of mine. His father then asked Michael for his keys, and without missing a single note, Michael handed his father the keys. The dream ended.

When I awoke I was completely elated from the experience of hearing such amazing music and from the feeling that Michael had made such progress. The next day, my mother telephoned and surprised me by saying that Michael's father had died just a few days before.

Dream 2

Recently, a colleague of mine in his late sixties was hit by a car and instantly died. Although I did not know him well, we had occasional conversations at lunch in the cafeteria of the school in which I taught and from which he had retired. He was a man highly devoted to helping the world improve. I heard of his death the day after it occurred, and that night, he appeared in a dream. He asked me sadly, "Am I really dead? Everyone says I am." I replied, "You were killed in an automobile accident." He then said, "How can I carry on all the important things I have been doing?" I said, "You will learn how to continue your work in a new way in your present state." He left, appearing very relieved and heartened.

A few days after having that dream, I went to his funeral—mainly out of curiosity. The person giving the eulogy kept saying how sad it was that the deceased was now separated from his family. I reflected that my dead colleague had made no mention of his wife and children but only his life's work. As we left, another teacher who had known him very well commented on how ironic the eulogy was, given that he had been estranged from his family for years and was totally involved in his work.

Dream 3

Years ago, I wanted to purchase a new computer. One of my colleagues suggested that I look into laptop computers. When I saw how expensive laptops were compared to desktop computers of the same power, I decided to get a desktop. A few months later, I had a dream that the laptop computers had been reduced to $19.95. I told my colleague of the dream. Periodically, he would jokingly ask me if I were going to get a laptop, and, each time, I would reply, "When they go down to $19.95."

The next September, a benefactor offered a $1000 rebate to any teacher who bought a computer. My colleague said, "If you buy a laptop now, it will cost you close to nothing." Shortly afterward, I bought a laptop computer with some extra memory. The amount I paid less $1000.00 came to $19.96—one cent more than in the dream.

Dream 4

This dream occurred on the morning of September 11, 2001, the morning that the World Trade Center was hit by jet airplanes: I was in my car, driving along a ramp which curved sharply upwards. I was very high up above the ground. I was starting to become terrified that my car would slip off the ramp, which was tilting sharply to the side. I carefully got out of my car, thinking, it's better to abandon my car than slip off and fall from this awful height. I found a stairway and got down to the street. I was very relieved to get away alive.

I then awoke to the clock radio and, shortly after, the news about the first plane hitting the Word Trade Center. Later, I viewed television videos of people jumping out of windows to their death. I then realized that I may have picked up the fear of those people and that that fear may have prompted my dream.

THE DIFFERENCE BETWEEN A DREAM, A HALLUCINATION, AND A VISION

Dreams, hallucinations, and visions all involve having an experience that does not occur in the physical word. In a dream, we experience a chain of events that we mistake for having occurred in the physical world. Because we are asleep (not in the physical world) at the time, our experience is not considered to be pathological although it involves a distortion. However, when we awaken, we realize our mistake. With training, dreams become more "lucid." That is, people who are dreaming become aware that they are not awake and can even control the experience or utilize it to soar into a higher plane as that experience evolves.

A hallucination is like a dream but occurs in the waking state. In a hallucination one should be in the physical world but is not. Thus, hallucinations are considered to be pathological. Hallucinations produced by drugs differ from those that are not. In the first case we can account for its reason whereas in the second case we cannot.

A vision is an experience that occurs while awake, most often during meditation. The person having the vision knows that his or her experience is not occurring in the physical world and is fully in touch with physical reality.

SOME DIFFERENCES BETWEEN PHILOSOPHY, RELIGION, SPIRITUAL TEACHINGS, AND SCIENCE

Philosophy

Philosophy is a method of logical inquiry into any and all manner of ideas. Philosophy is the application of clear and analytical thinking to unscrambling the complexities of problems that are very difficult for the mind to encompass. Philosophy can be applied to ethics, science, metaphysics, religion, study of the mind, etc. In China, Buddhism and Daoism are regarded as both philosophies and religions. As philosophies, Buddhism and Daoism are totally compatible with each other and with religions. Religions, on the other hand, tend not to be compatible with each other; namely, it is not likely for a person to be a Catholic and a Jew at the same time.

Religion

Imagine a culture in which children are fed insects at an early age. Similarly, imagine another culture in which children are taught not to eat insects. The mouth of a person who grew up in the first culture might water upon seeing an insect, whereas a person who grew up in the second culture might experience revulsion at the mere sight of an insect and would certainly be disgusted at the sight of someone eating one. Were a person of the non-bug-eating culture to be invited to dinner by a person of the bug-eating one, there well might be a problem. This analogy applies to religion. At early ages, children of each religion are taught precepts that are different from those taught to children of other religions. Those espousing each religion find it hard to accept the beliefs of those of another religion.

A hallmark of religion is not to question the "word of God," each different version of which is represented in the Old Testament, New Testament, Koran, etc. Some religions actually punish, excommunicate, or consider to be dead those who break the tenets of their religion. There is no possibility for a member of a religion to proclaim that God does not exist and still be accepted as a member of that religion by its most orthodox members.

Spiritual Teachings

Spiritual teachings, on the other hand, foster individual development. Such teachings cultivate a questioning attitude and emphasize discarding or at least putting into perspective one's preprogrammed ideas and "knowledge." In spiritual teachings, nothing is sacred other than being in harmony with the Universe. The precepts of such harmony are not indoctrinated but are experienced first hand through meditation and introspection.

Science

Science is similar in some ways to spiritual teachings except that the language of science is mathematics. That is, if an idea is incapable of being put into numerical terms, the knowledge such ideas express is considered to be on a low level. Scientific statements that do not predict or explain are considered to be undependable. Moreover, statements whose truth or falsity have no way of being tested are considered to be scientifically meaningless and not in the domain of science. Such statements are rejected by scientists as having no scientific validity. This principle is called *the verifiability theory of meaning.*

One of the tenets of science is to reject old ideas as new information becomes validated—not right away or frivolously but eventually as the strength of evidence mounts. The great discoveries in science, such as in the areas of astronomy, quantum mechanics, and relativity, all required discarding prior ideas and psychological attachments in favor of new ones for which overwhelming evidence was found.

Whereas blind acceptance is antithetical to scientific inquiry, unfortunately most people rely on "experts" for scientific truth. Primary and secondary schools do not teach students to understand, analyze, compare, remember, interpret, or logically apply scientific information. Most people learn science by rote—if they learn any science at all. The result is that, for many people, science is a religion.

SOME QUESTIONS AND ANSWERS

The following is an almost verbatim transcript of answers I gave to questions asked by my students at Fieldston H.S. on November 24, 1999.

1. What is the meaning of life?

This subject is very important for us to consider because it affects our entire approach to everything we do and say. My thinking on this subject was greatly influenced by a book, *On Being Human*, by Ashley Montagu.[88] In that book Montagu presents the following way of looking at things: One idea that may seem to follow from looking at the different living creatures is that the most aggressive and strongest life forms win out by devouring the weaker ones ("tooth-and-claw theory"). However, if we follow the evolution of life from its beginning, we see that life forms have developed first as individual cells, which had no connection with each other except when propagation was required (if you watch amoebas and paramecium under a microscope, you will observe them to occasionally group together in a huge mound to exchange genetic material). As time went on, life forms began to consist of multiple cells, all existing harmoniously. Today, we are examples of living structures comprising many different organs consisting of highly specialized cells. We have skin cells,

---

88. Ashley Montagu, *On Being Human*, Hawthorn Books, Inc., New York, 1966.

bone cells, mucus membrane cells, blood cells (if you can call them cells), nerve cells, cells of reception of temperature, pressure, smell, taste, and vibration, etc. All of these cells must be in harmony with each other for us to survive as individuals. Moreover, all our glands and organs must likewise be in harmony. Whereas some complex animals just lay eggs and do not care for or rear their young, many life forms bring up their offspring. Many life forms such as bees, ants, and humans have complex societies wherein individuals take on special functions such as teachers and garbage collectors so that society can function. If we look around, we can see strife and chaos, but if we were to be really objective, we would see tremendous harmony between individuals. When you're in your car, you may feel that people are going too fast or slow, cutting you off, or following too close, but if you view traffic from a helicopter, you'd be amazed at how harmoniously traffic flows.

The meaning of life is that we are consciousnesses, placed in these bodies for on the order of one-hundred years, here to use our creative intelligence to produce harmony. We are also here to grow by observing the harmony all around us, especially as expressed in nature. Our consciousnesses existed long before they came into these bodies and will continue to exist long after. This is not really my own idea but what I have learned from studying meditation and reading books on metaphysics. Of course, I would not be repeating it if I did not accept the truth of it and live it from day to day. Much of this knowledge is thousands of years old and understood by many people in the world. Many books contain this knowledge, but they are not read by many. Some of these books are very hard to understand. It might take years to understand just one page. In this part of the world our emphasis has been on developing material things and making money rather than on spiritual development. We have ignored this knowledge even though it is readily available. We have cellular telephones, the Internet, etc., and knowledge from all over the world can be ours for the asking. Everywhere, there are spiritual teachers who have only a few students. At this time, when we have access to knowledge from all parts of the world and from far into the past, most people are oblivious. Not everyone, though.

2. How old are our consciousnesses? Are they as old as the earth?

Our consciousnesses have existed long before they came into these bodies and will continue long after the body has died. Try to think of when your consciousness began. Did it begin when you were born? Probably not. Did it begin when the sperm met the egg? The Buddhists believe that the consciousness becomes attracted to the fetus as it starts to develop and makes a stronger and stronger connection as the fetus grows. By the time the child is born, there is a fairly strong connection. During the individual's lifetime the connection becomes very strong, and then as the individual moves toward the end of his life, it weakens again, as it should.

With regard to the age of our consciousness, the concept of time may well be meaningless when it comes to a realm that is non-physical. In the physical world, time has meaning, but that is not the only realm. This assertion is mentioned in a number of books on metaphysics. Once, during meditation, I had the distinct perception that it made sense for there to be a realm in which time was not a factor.

3. How can consciousness be non-physical?

Because we are in the physical world, sense data comes in very strongly through our physical senses of touch, sight, hearing, smell, etc. This sense data tends to mask awareness of other planes, and we tend to think that the physical world is the only real world. When we are asleep or in a state of meditation, we disregard input from our senses, and awareness of what enters from other realms is heightened. If we have a dream, when we wake up, we say, "That really didn't happen—it was a dream." However, we did have an experience, but because we believe that the physical world encompasses all of reality, we misinterpret what we experienced. Even during the dream, untrained people interpret their experiences through the same wrong belief that the physical world is the only world. That's one reason why people who are interested in spiritual development do meditation—so that they can subdue what comes in through the senses and experience that which is not in the physical world.

4. Why do we come into these bodies?

Some books on metaphysics say that all of us here in the physical plane are missing some basic elements in our development, which, if we don't remedy will cause us to be here indefinitely. We come here to grow spiritually and to develop an increased understanding of harmony as expressed in nature. Most of us do not do that. We think we are here just to enjoy ourselves and have our senses stimulated by food, entertainment, and sex. If not placed in this stringent physical world, some of us would not progress. The physical world is so stringent that if you so much as hold a piece of paper the wrong way you can get a paper cut that affects your whole day.

5. If there were a giant computer, would it have a consciousness?

This concept stems from the idea scientists have that consciousness and brain are the same. They are not the same because consciousness, which is non-physical, can exist without a brain, which is physical. It seems unlikely that a computer can have consciousness. A computer is totally preprogrammed. It has no free will. It does only that which is programmed into it's circuits and no more. There would be no reason for a consciousness to reside in a computer, which is totally preprogrammed and affords no opportunity for its spiritual growth.

Some people will say that each person is like a complex computer. They say that we may think we have free will, but we really don't. They say that everything we do and say is preprogrammed. And, to be sure, that is true for most people. Because many people focus their energies on the pursuit of money, entertainment, and pleasures of the senses, they may never achieve free will and a knowledge of why they are here. However, just because they do not experience free will, that does not mean that free will does not exist. That is the purpose of meditation—to transcend the preprogrammed thinking we all have. If you study meditation or a meditative art such as Yoga or Taiji, you will find that you do have free will.

6. Do animals have consciousness? If so, is an animal's consciousness less developed than that of a human?

It is clear from observing animals that they have consciousness and free will, just as do other people. Anyone who has had a pet knows that animals have feelings, emotions, and consciousness. The hormones associated with the various emotions are the same in animals as humans. That is why people who are deficient in certain hormones such as thyroid, can be given animal hormones as replacement (many of these hormones now can be synthesized).

An animal's consciousness would appear to be less developed than those in humans, but it may be that a developed consciousness may find its way into an animal. According to some metaphysical teachings, consciousness can reside in a person, an animal, or even a tree. It is hard to imagine consciousness residing in inanimate, non-living objects like rocks. However, it may be that life goes way beyond our concept of it. Perhaps there is life in the center of the earth or inside the sun. Of course, that kind of life would be very different from ours. Just as our bodies are made up of water, oxygen, and minerals characteristic of our environment, life in the center of the sun would similarly be made up of the hot gasses and plasma there.

7. How do I know that I have a consciousness? You must define it if we are going to talk about it in any meaningful way.

A few years ago I was listening to an interview with a famous psychologist on my car radio. He said that those in his field have recently come to realize that no further progress can be made without defining consciousness. He went on to say that another psychologist had, over the past five years, read everything written about consciousness and had formulated a definition. Not wanting to miss hearing this definition, I pulled onto the shoulder of the road and listened intently. The definition was, "Consciousness is the way the mind views the world." My first thought was that it would take more than a lifetime to even scratch the surface of everything written about consciousness. Much of what is written is in obscure languages and very difficult to translate into English. Also, the definition was circular. I then asked myself how *I* would define consciousness. The conclusion I came to is similar to that of physicists when presented with the problem of defining time.

If you look up the word *time* in a dictionary, you will find that it is defined in terms of sequences of events. If you look up the word *sequence*, it will involve *time*, and so on. Even though the definition of time is problematic, we, nevertheless, feel that we know what time is and understand it.

Physicists deal with this problem as follows: Quantities such as speed, force, acceleration, momentum, energy, etc., need to be defined mathematically and non-circularly in terms of other quantities. However, at some point, there remain a small number of what are called *fundamental quantities* that cannot be defined in terms of any other quantities without circularity. Because physics is a science that relates to the physical world, it must be grounded, that is, connected somehow to the physical world. Physicists decided that a satisfactory way of defining the three fundamental quantities, namely, time, length, and mass, is to say that these quantities are defined in the way they are measured. In that way, the fundamental quantities are defined in a way that connects them directly to the physical world. Physicists say that the "fundamental quantities" time, length, and mass are defined "operationally."

I reasoned as follows: Just as physics is a science pertaining to the physical world, psychology is a science that pertains to the mental world. Just as physics must be tied to the physical world through definitions directly connecting quantities with the physical world, psychology must tie basic quantities to the mental world. The fact is that if there is such a thing as consciousness (if not, why would we be trying to define it?), we all have it and experience it constantly. Thus, consciousness is a perfect concept to define "operationally." That is, we should not try to define it in terms of anything other than our own experience and leave it at that.

Each of us has a consciousness. If anyone says, "I don't know what consciousness is," it is really almost impossible to explain it to him.

8. What is wrong with doing things that make us happy? It doesn't sound like you'd be very happy pursuing a life devoted to spiritual growth.

Life is more than eating, sleeping, entertainment, and fulfilling sexual needs, though these activities certainly have their place. To most people, happiness is having fun and being distracted from the emptiness of their lives. Such people are preprogrammed, have little or no free will, and experience periodic cycles of happiness and despair. Because they haven't the slightest idea of why they are here, their lives consist of pursuing money, entertainment, and pleasures of the senses. But on one level, deep down, they recognize that their lives are not fulfilling their purpose for being here, namely, to grow and help others grow. They feel a void but mistakenly try to fill that void with the same things but with more intensity. They eat food that is so spicy that it burns their tongue and digestive tract. They over-indulge in sex, over-eat to the point of extreme obesity, listen to music that is so loud that it actually damages their hearing, and, in many cases, turn to drugs to achieve a heightened experience. Once you recognize your reason for being here and work to fulfill it, there is a long-term sense of fulfillment that transcends happiness, which is fleeting.

9. It sounds like it is very hard to change the emphasis from getting pleasure from life to fulfillment.

It's very easy and natural. What's hard is trying to go against nature's laws—to be out of harmony with your purpose for being here.

13

Further Self-Development Through Teaching Taiji: Practical Suggestions

Teaching is important for accelerating self-development and progress in Taiji. Teaching is a natural way of sharing something that you love. Teaching challenges your knowledge and skill and is crucial for the development and expansion of the art you teach.

WHEN ARE YOU READY TO TEACH YOUR OWN CLASSES?

Getting permission from your teacher beforehand is always best. Do not feel that you have to have mastered Taiji in order to teach it; when you begin teaching, enthusiasm can make up for some lack of knowledge and Taiji ability. Of course, you must always be open about your limitations of knowledge and skill. Such openness is equally important when you become established as a master teacher.

When I had been studying Taiji for three years with Zheng Manqing, I interviewed for a job teaching science and other subjects at an alternative high school. During the interview, I was asked what alternative topics I could teach. One of the first topics I thought of was Taiji. It never occurred to me to ask permission from Zheng to teach Taiji.

At Zheng's school, Shr Jung Center for Culture and the Arts, at 87 Bowery, in Chinatown New York City, I naively mentioned to one of the senior students, Lou Kleinsmith, about my commitment to teach Taiji. To my amazement Kleinsmith was horrified and immediately brought me to Professor Zheng. Some of the other senior students were also present. To the senior students' surprise, when Zheng heard that a "beginning" student was going to teach, he calmly gave his permission and assigned me to assist teaching part of Tam Gibbs' class at the school. Zheng also had Gibbs mentor me so that I would be ready to teach at the alternative school by September. I was elated, for teaching at Zheng's school was an honor and something I had hoped to be able to do at some point.

During a class I was leading, Gibbs would correct my egregious mistakes in front of the students, which was very embarrassing. Soon, I lost my embarrassment and began to value his corrections. I learned a lot from Tam about teaching, both during and after class, when we discussed errors in my teaching and movements. By September, I felt much more ready to teach on my own.

After a month or two of teaching on my own, another senior student, Maggie Newman, visited my class. I was very honored by her offer to come. Later, I realized that her visit must have been arranged by Zheng, partly as a back-up and partly to make sure that I was not doing something wrong.

About a year or so after I began teaching on my own, I received a telephone call from a senior student, who asked me if I would be willing to take over an ongoing class. This class was fairly close to where I lived and had been taught by a classmate who was moving out of the area. I jumped at the opportunity. I soon realized that in Taiji, whereas there are no belts as in Karate, there are other ways that a student's progress is acknowledged. Being given a class to teach is one of those ways.

STARTING OUT TEACHING

Teaching at a Yoga or Martial-Arts Center

At the beginning, finding your own space and starting your own classes can be quite difficult. Those who run Yoga and martial-arts centers usually have high rents and seek ways to make money during off hours. They also want to expand their offerings. It is my experience that such centers tend not to be able to attract sufficient Taiji students to be able to pay you a substantial amount for your teaching. At the same time, their need to maintain a reputation for quality teaching will rule out accepting any other than a veteran teacher. Therefore, trying to teach in such a center may not be the best idea for a beginning teacher. Adult-education programs tend to be a better alternative.

Teaching in an Adult-Education Program

Starting an evening class in an ongoing adult-education program at a public school or a community center has both advantages and disadvantages. One advantage is that some of the students will eventually become your own and stay with you for years. Unfortunately, my experience over the past three decades is that administrators of adult-education programs can sometimes be inflexible and unrealistic and have little idea of the problems with starting a Taiji class and then sustaining it. For example, a typical series will run for eight or ten weeks. When the session ends, some students will want to continue, but classes are then suspended for months. Usually, the administrator will mistakenly expect that these same students will return after that lapse and become indignant if you continue to teach these students on your own, which is really the responsible thing to do.

Therefore, it is important to achieve a mutual understanding of these matters at the outset. It is best to avoid teaching in programs where there is no provision for students to continue without interruption, either in the adult-education program or privately when the series ends.

Another issue is that adult-education-program administrators sometimes want the fees students pay to be unreasonably low, which means that your remuneration, which is usually based on enrollment, can be minimal. If the session is renewed, the inevitable drop-off in attendance will further reduce your remuneration.

Finally, some administrators expect that, should the session be renewed, new students will be able to attend and be taught along with the older ones. Dealing with multiple levels of ability without help from advanced students can be difficult for a beginning teacher, and this difficulty should be considered before agreeing to teach on such a basis.

Teaching at a Fitness Club

I have taught at three fitness clubs, two of which provided a very good experience. The third club was very swanky and was characterized by extremely loud music from aerobics classes, unwillingness to provide a suitably large space, lack of respect, low salary, and lack of job security.

Space Requirements

The following formula for determining how much space is needed has proved to be reliable: 100 square feet of floor space plus an additional 30 square feet per student. A wooden or rug-covered floor and mirrors on a wall are desirable but not necessary.

TEACHING ON YOUR OWN

Finding a Space in Which to Teach

Using your house as a studio for your own practice is fine, and expenses from such use may be used as a deduction against your earnings. However, teaching classes in your home can be problematic. I used to hold classes in my home successfully for years without any problem, but in today's litigious world, I minimize that use only to occaisionally teaching several students I know well.

Possibilities for rental space are houses of worship, temporarily empty store fronts, businesses with space to rent during off hours, dance studios, Yoga and martial-arts schools, and even schools during evenings. When I searched for a space years ago, I found that rental fees ranged from "pay whatever you can" to more than I could hope to make from my students. Because of the uncertain nature of whether classes will succeed, it is better to pay by the hour than by the month or year.

Once you find a suitable space, it is important to be responsible. Make sure that you and your students leave no mess, close windows and turn off heat and lights when leaving, and report and offer to pay for or personally repair any damage you or your students do. Because I have the skill to do so, I have done several repairs to generally improve the space that I rent.

Publicity

Once you have secured a space, one of the best ways to start a new class is to give a "demonstration." You will need to create a poster, which should have a picture of yourself; the date, time, and place of the demonstration; the words *no charge*; a short description of Taiji; a blurb about yourself containing what you have studied plus other accomplishments; and a telephone number that people can call for information. Include the address of your web site if you have one. It is good to have a series of "tear-offs" containing essential information at the bottom of your poster.

If the class is sponsored by a fitness club or an adult-education program, they will usually publicize the demonstration, but supplying them with a poster will facilitate things and head off their creating a poster that may have inappropriate wording, clip-art, and general appearance. If you are starting a class on your own, you will need to put up posters in supermarkets, health-food stores, libraries, and other places that have bulletin boards. Some newspapers will print a blurb in their "Events" section without charge. An advertisement appearing a week before in a local newspaper or similar publication is not costly and can be of value. It is good to assemble a list of interested people and send out an announcement several weeks in advance by mail or email. The day of the week and starting time of the demonstration should be the same as that of the class you intend to give.

The demonstration should include a brief description of Taiji and its basic principles, doing a section of the form alone or with your students, and teaching several movements to those attending. After the demonstration, you (or, preferably, one of your students) should give information about the upcoming classes and sign up interested people.

Talking to Potential Students on the Telephone

It is my experience and also that of other teachers that few people who call actually come to a class. People call for many reasons. Some callers are bored and just want to talk to someone. Others are actually interested in starting an exercise program but do not yet know which. Still others have called so many teachers of Taiji and similar arts that they can't even remember all the people to whom they have spoken. I occasionally get calls from people who have or who know others who have serious diseases and desperately want to explore alternative solutions. Even some of those who call you in earnest may not have the same enthusiasm a few days later. So do not become discouraged or wonder what you said wrong when people fail to show up.

It is important not to talk on the telephone too long. After the standard questions have been answered, I say, "Are there any other questions?" If none, I say, "I'm looking forward to meeting you on Saturday," which is a nice way of ending the conversation.

Yellow Pages Listing

There is no specific "Yellow Pages" listing for Taiji. The listing must be under "Karate & Other Martial Arts." I have tried such a listing twice. Both times, the only responses I received were those from people asking my advice about enrolling their young children in Karate and Tae Kwon

Do classes. Sometimes I was on the telephone for an extended period of time, politely listening to questions and giving advice.

Maintaining a Web Page

Make sure that your web page is user and search-engine friendly. Beware of including jazzy, flashy, distractions such as rotating Taiji symbols, flashing headlines, etc. These gimmicks are antithetical to the Taiji principle of non-action and can take a long time for visitors to download.

> *Any intelligent fool can make things bigger, more complex, and more violent. It takes a touch of genius—and a lot of courage—to move in the opposite direction.*
>
> —Albert Einstein

Include information on the time and place of each class, whether beginners are welcome to start at any time, and how to get there from different directions. There should be information about Taiji in general, the nature of your classes, and your credentials (academic degrees, the extent of your Taiji training, and the teachers with whom you have studied). There should also be an email address or telephone number so that potential students can reach you. It is also valuable to provide information that goes beyond you and your classes. The most-trafficked Taiji websites have genealogies, information on famous masters, links to other teachers' sites, philosophy, and provisions for practitioner-intercommunication.

The Best Times to Start a New Class

I have noticed that people are most interested in starting a constructive activity in early September and January. Apparently New Year's Eve for many people is a "day of atonement." After realizing that another year has passed unproductively and with last year's resolutions unfulfilled, many people make resolutions for the next year. Therefore, in January, many people tend to be more receptive to starting Taiji.

WHOM SHOULD YOU TEACH?

Teaching Youngsters

The youngest student I ever taught was a boy, nine years of age. When I expressed my doubt about the appropriateness of someone so young studying Taiji, I was informed that he had a black belt in Judo and knew what he was getting into. He came to all classes of the ten-week series but acted like a kid of his age, with wandering attentiveness and a lack of interest in the principles. However, he perked up whenever I demonstrated martial applications. He did not continue past the first ten-week series.

I have had success with a few twelve-year-olds, but most children of that age are too young to study Taiji. Those over 16 years of age are quite receptive to learning Taiji and love it. I taught Taiji successfully as an extra-curricular activity and as a physical education elective at Fieldston High School for 23 years. Some of these students continued their study of Taiji afterward, in college. Some others subsequently took up the study of other martial arts.

Teaching the Elderly

Teaching seniors can been an extremely satisfying experience. Being in the presence of those with more life experience can enhance your perspective. Whereas seniors tend not to practice on their own and many have poor retention of the movements, all of them benefit in their own ways. A lot of patience is needed in repeatedly going over movements, but, overall, the experience pays off. Every now and then, an elderly student will say something heartening such as, "I used to fall frequently, but I have not fallen once since starting Taiji."

It is important to recognize that some seniors cannot stand for a long period of time. Therefore, meditative stretching on the floor is usually appreciated and of much benefit. Also, certain exercises can be done while sitting. The following balance exercise is valuable: Stand on one leg and slowly and gently move the other leg in every possible direction. Keep an awareness that the weight distribution of the weighted foot is centered on the center of that foot and that the center of mass of the body also stays directly over the center of the weighted foot.

Teaching Those Who Have Studied With Other Teachers

Every now and then, those with previous training come to my classes. I will usually ask such students to show me their movements. Before giving any corrections, the most important thing you can do is to compliment that student and, if possible his/her teacher. If a student has previously studied Taiji and is now continuing to study, that in itself demonstrates a laudable interest. The student has already put in a certain amount of work and practice, which should be recognized.

Be careful not to succumb to an impulse to judge that student's teacher; the student may not represent what the teacher taught or it might unnecessarily offend the student and will put you in a bad light.

Teaching Other Taiji Teachers

There is a tendency not to share your knowledge and teaching methods with those who might compete with you. On the other hand, such sharing enables the art to develop and spreads the benefit of your knowledge to more people. Also, collegial sharing accelerates your own growth in Taiji.

TEACHING-METHODS AND CLASS MANAGEMENT

You may get more students in teaching superficially or by rote, but you will be cheating your students, and your self-development dividends will be less. Teaching from principles rather than by rote will attract the kind of student who will challenge you productively with thoughtful questions that refine your understanding.

Starting Off a New Student or Group

At the beginning of the first class, I ask if students have any prior experience with Taiji. Knowing the depth of students' prior experience helps to calibrate the level on which I will teach. If there are some students with prior experience, I still teach on a beginning level but add a few advanced concepts. During the class, I teach only several movements of the form but make sure that beginners understand that their job is to own the movements so that they can practice on their own without needing to follow others.

At the end of the first class, I say, "Practice every day. If you forget a movement, make something up. Even if you are doing it incorrectly, next class you will immediately change and get it right. Otherwise, what you learned will evaporate, and we will have to start afresh."

Absorbing Beginners in an Ongoing Class Versus Starting a New Homogenous Class

For quite a few years I prohibited beginners from entering an ongoing class. I lost potential students that way. People would call me, enthusiastic about starting. I would take their names and telephone numbers, saying that I would call them when the next beginners' class started. When I called them a month or so later, their interest had usually evaporated. Moreover, students in an all-beginners' class have little idea of the depth of the art or the skill level of the teacher. As a result, they get easily discouraged, tend not to practice, and do not have much reverence for what they are taught.

I saw that other Taiji and other martial arts teachers with whom I have studied let beginners start at any time. These beginners made fast progress because they were exposed to a higher level of teaching and could observe and be inspired by more-advanced students. Therefore, I decided to let new students into an ongoing class. It took a while to become proficient in adding new students, but it was worth the additional effort. For example, one dividend is that, after class, a new student will sometimes get into a conversation with an advanced student, who will say something encouraging to the newcomer. All of these factors are reasons to learn to naturally absorb beginners into an ongoing class.

Adding beginners requires creativity because every situation is different. What I do is let the beginner follow along for the first class. I tell the beginner not to worry so much about hands but pay attention mostly to the placement, angling, and relative weight distribution of the feet.

If the other students are not far along, for the first or several subsequent classes, I may go over the first few moves with everybody. Ideally, the beginner will be concentrating on the bare bones of the move, and the other students will be getting some new slant or reviewing a concept to which they have been previously exposed but have not completely mastered. After a while I tell the beginner, "Practice on your own while I work with the rest of the class." Periodically, I repeat that process.

Or, I may teach everyone awhile, with the beginner following along. Then I give the class something to work on by themselves or in groups. That frees me to teach the beginner. After a while, I tell the beginner,

"Practice on your own while I work with the rest of the class." I alternate that way, as appropriate.

Having More-Advanced Students Assist in Teaching

If one of my students is sufficiently advanced, I let that student work with one or more beginners, or I work with the beginners myself and have the advanced student lead or even teach the rest of the class. At the half point, I swap roles with the advanced student.

As time goes by, I have more students who can assist me in teaching, which makes absorbing a beginner easier. Also, the students who are teaching tend to do a good job, get a lot out of it, and usually enjoy doing it. Rotating the use of advanced students reduces the time they miss from their instruction.

Some teachers with whom I have studied let new students go for the first few months before providing them with any individualized instruction. I do not like that method at all.

Because of the academic and analytical way that I teach Taiji, I seem to get many students who are fairly intellectual, have the skills to eventually assist me in teaching, and are eager to teach. However, I always feel out a student whom I want to assist me. If I see any reluctance, I find another student or alternative.

Teaching a New Movement

One aspect of the balance of yin and yang (passive and active, respectively,) in teaching is as follows: The teacher shows a new movement, instructing students to watch but not imitate the movement. After showing a movement several times and pointing out the "landmarks," the teacher then allows the students to follow along several times. Next, the teacher instructs students to practice that movement on their own awhile. The whole process is then repeated. Watching the teacher without doing any movement inculcates the ability to observe and form a mental image of the important features and helps students ascertain whether or not the movement is "owned."

Initial Student Enthusiasm

There is often an inverse relationship between students' initial enthusiasm and the length of time that they will pursue the study of Taiji. Students who say things like "I know I will do this for the rest of my life" will often drop out very quickly. One reason may be that love at first sight is often an infatuation that evaporates once the student realizes that daily solo practice is necessary for progress. On the other hand, when a student exercises skepticism and reservation, that student's love for Taiji is more apt to be real and, therefore, long-lived.

Asking Students Questions in Class

Notice how engaged and alert you become when someone asks you a question. One of the basic principles of teaching any subject matter is to ask students questions. Then give them time to think. In most academic classes, the first person to raise his/her hand gets called on, which shuts off the thought processes of all the other students who need to give a bit more thought to the question. Some students might not have even heard the question. Therefore, it is good not to call on the first students who raise their hands but allow time for others to process the question.

Reinforcement of Concepts Taught and Class-to-Class Continuity

Few students are able to either immediately learn a new concept or follow it up with practice and questions later on. Therefore, it is of much value to repeat showing a particular way of moving or of explaining a particular concept from class to class. If possible, occasionally have a senior student come up to the front of the class to give his/her version. Also, it is good for the teacher to remember what was taught in a class and review it at some point in the next class. At the end of a class, it is very helpful to students to review the important points of a class and remind them to practice and reflect on them.

Formal or Informal Classes?

You can be as formal as you want. It is totally up to you. In some classes, the teacher is on a first-name basis, students and teacher wear whatever clothing they desire, and the teaching space has no tapestries or pictures. In other classes, the teacher is addressed as *Sifu*, and students are required to wear a specified uniform or only certain color combinations, sashes, and patches. Tapestries, calligraphy, sayings, and pictures of the grandmaster hang from the wall of the teaching space.

Doing Warm-Up/Stretching/Qigong in Class?

Many Taiji instructors start with the form without prior warm-up, stretching, or Qigong exercises. I have found that leading a short-but-thorough warm-up followed by meditative stretching on mats on the floor (see Chapter 6) is of much value. After that, we do about 10–20 minutes of Qigong. Finally, all students do the first section of the form, led by me or one of my senior students. Then we break up into groups by level so that each student can get personalized instruction.

Here are the advantages of doing an initial warm-up, meditative stretching, and Qigong: (1) Students like it—some elderly students come just for that part of the class. (2) It helps students and teacher achieve a relaxed state much sooner than doing Taiji movements for the same amount of time. (3) It allows students to experience important facets of Taiji such as song, use of muscular extension, and qi much earlier than they would while concentrating on learning movements, balance, stepping, etc.

Treatment of Guests

Guests should be treated appropriately, whether potential students or a student's friends. When guests come, at first opportunity, I introduce myself, shake hands, and welcome them to the class. At the end of the class, I go over to any guests and thank them for coming. I also ask, "Do you have any observations?"

Dealing with Disruptions to Classes

Noise. The first time that I taught at an adult-education center, the initial class was held in one half of a large room separated by a thin partition. A tap-dance class was in the other half. The noise was so loud that my students could barely hear me. Nevertheless, I continued with the class. Pretty soon, our concentration was sufficient to minimize the effect of the noise. Of course, the noise problem was corrected after the first class. In general, unless the noise is so loud that it is impossible to concentrate, it is a good exercise to disregard it and instruct students to do the same.

Holidays. Any break in continuity of class time creates a loss of some students, but a break involving two or more classes in a row can be devastating. My policy is not to suspend class unless it is on Christmas Day. A few times, we had class on New Year's Eve. Amazingly attendance was 100%, and it was a memorable experience to do meditative movement while everyone else was preparing for a lively evening.

Having Students Work in Pairs

I have found it valuable to present a concept in detail, answer questions, and then pair students off. Some exercises require both people to work together simultaneously, and others require one student to do movements while the other observes and makes constructive criticisms. Still other exercises require some physical contact. In all cases, it is important to provide sufficient time for students to swap roles and to change partners. When there is an odd number of students, I work with the odd student, or, should I need to go to the other groups, I form a three-person group.

Showing Self-Defense Applications of Movements

Even though I do not emphasize self-defense in the classes that I teach, I feel that it is good to show the applications with which I am familiar. Seeing the applications of a movement helps students to remember that movement better and do it more correctly. Doing movement in agreement with the self-defense principles almost always enhances the health and self-development aspects.

Of course, showing self-defense applications requires another person. Correctly choosing that person is critical. Choosing the wrong person to use to demonstrate applications can result in your appearing inept. Those viewing will usually not realize that punches and kicks that have no intention or are out of range need not be defended against and are awkward to try to pretend to counter. Attacks must be slow and definite, and the attacker must be willing to act the part; namely, if what, on the street, would be a hard strike to the head is employed without contact in class, the recipient must pretend that the effect of that strike is real. Just because students have studied martial arts before does not mean that they will be good partners for demonstrating self-defense applications. Other students will not necessarily want to be the recipient of simulated strikes, kicks, etc., even if no harm is done to them. Also, it should be explained that it is inappropriate for a student to try to compete with the teacher at a time when such movements are being shown purely for instruction.

Answering Questions in Class

Questions range from where to step in a given movement to complex issues such as breathing, qi, yin and yang, etc. I make it a rule to do the following three things when answering questions:

1. I always admit when I do not know the answer, and I am honest about revealing the limits of my knowledge and skill. To do otherwise would hamper both my progress and that of my students. When a student asks me a question that I cannot answer or have difficulty in answering, I consider it an opportunity for my development.

2. I always try to answer a question from principles—even when the question is simply about the placement of a foot.

3. I never disparage any question, and I commend the student for asking it. If a student asks a question that someone has already asked, I answer the question in a new way. Making students feel foolish for asking questions stunts their growth and discourages others from asking questions.

When a student asks the same question more than once, I assume that a second, new answer is required and take that as an opportunity to refine my explanation, not only for that student but for everyone, including myself. In that vein, I once asked my teacher Harvey Sober a question, to which he humorously replied, "You asked that question a few months ago." I replied, "I just wanted to get a second opinion." Everyone in the class knew that Sober's answer would have a new dimension, and, of course, it did.

Mistakes

Mistakes are for learning. Everyone makes mistakes. It is impossible to learn without them. The best policy is not to hide mistakes but use them for self-improvement and for teaching your students.

Attempting to convince your students that you never make mistakes is bad for them and bad for you. Each time you hide your own mistakes from your students you deprive them of one of the best opportunities for learning. True, some students will be disappointed that you are not perfect, but they are free to seek a "perfect master." The others, who are there to learn, will admire your honesty and come away with an enhanced understanding. Moreover, you will be inculcating similar behavior in them.

When I taught physics, I found that the most exciting moments for my students and myself were when I made an error in doing a problem at the blackboard. Either a student or I would discover that an error had been made, and then finding the mistake became an exciting adventure. When a student or I found the error, there would be an exuberance unmatched by other learning situations. If I found the error first, I would ask the class if I should tell them. Often, they preferred to continue to devote more thought in class or at home.

Releasing Students

At a certain point, students need to make a change in teacher or in the art they are studying. It is essential to release such students gracefully.

Expelling Students (Mentally)

In over three decades of teaching, I have only had several students whom I dismissed. None of these students realized that I had taken an active part in their dismissal because it was done mentally.

The following is an example of mentally influencing a desired outcome: I did not want to teach a particular session of a beginner's class that I had periodically taught for many years. Several months before the session was slated to start, I set my mind that it would not go. A week before the class was scheduled to start, the perplexed director of the program called me, apologetically explaining that no one had registered for my course.

Competitors

The main competitors are fitness clubs, Yoga, Pilates, Tae Kwon Do, and other movement arts that have recently become popular. Those who are already engaged in these activities are less likely to take on an additional activity in a different location. Competitors can be other Taiji teachers, some of whom can be your colleagues, classmates, teachers, or even your own students.

If you do not teach Taiji as your main livelihood, it is easier to tell new students, who come from large distances, of qualified teachers much closer to them. Another possibility is referring students to other arts that would be more suitable for them. You may lose a few students this way, but it might be that other teachers will reciprocate, which has been my experience. It is especially gratifying to have the experience of telling a student about a closer teacher and have that student decide to stay with you.

Teaching Private Classes

Whereas I am willing to teach private classes when I have the time, I am usually reluctant to do so. Such classes tend to be intense and draining and much less stimulating to teach than a class with a many students. Also, I want what I say to go out to as many people as possible. For these reasons, if I am going to teach a private class, I stipulate that whatever the length of the class, I will prorate the hourly rate. Then I can let the class end when it is appropriate to do so—usually after about a half an hour.

There is a tendency for private students to engage you in friendly conversation or even questions about Taiji after the class ends, which can be problematic if your time is limited. Sometimes, it is necessary to find a way to have a definite ending to a class without being abrupt.

Size of Classes

From the point of view of excitement in teaching and community of learning, large classes are definitely preferable. Also, a new class will usually decrease in size, so it is good to start large. However, when the class is too large (more than twenty students), it becomes difficult or even impossible to correct students individually. Then, when possible, it is advantageous to have your more-advanced students come to help out. For example, a student who has completed the form and has received substantial corrections can lead the class. That student can be instructed to stop and hold a particular posture while you correct students in the class. Or, that student can lead the entire form or a section of it while you observe those doing the form—leader included—and make corrections afterward.

When a class becomes so small that continuing is not cost effective or stimulating to teacher or students, I personally feel an obligation to try to make some arrangement that allows the remaining students to continue. For example, several small classes can be amalgamated, or students can be invited to come to an ongoing class that can accommodate them. As a last resort, students can be advised to study with another qualified teacher.

STUDENT POSITIONING

Even in a large room, Taiji students feel obligated to give the teacher half of the space. To make things worse, students tend to arrange themselves in rows rather than stagger their positions. The teacher then needs to encourage students to optimize the use of space.

The teacher also should encourage students to occasionally change their habitual locations when doing the form together in class. Students and teacher then view each other's movement from new lines of sight. The teacher can then provide new corrections, and students can ask new questions.

Additionally, students should be made aware not to block the view of a classmate or guest during times when the class forms a circle around the teacher.

Humor

I have been a student of quite a few arts and sciences and can say that the classes that involved humor were the most enjoyable and resulted in the most retention. Classes in which no humor or light-heartedness occur tend to be dry and even boring. Laughter is relaxing, cultivates student-teacher and student-student bonds, and has an uplifting, buoyant effect. It is, of course, inappropriate to turn Taiji class into a comedy routine or to feel pressured to make your students laugh, but the effectiveness and appropriateness of humor, naturally expressed, cannot be overemphasized.

Correcting Students

It is hard to predict what region of the body to which a student might have such a strong emotional attachment that it is off grounds to even refer to—let alone touch. It always is good to approach correcting students by sensing their degree of receptivity. Correcting students by touching them should be done cautiously, and for some students, not at all.

Teaching Qi to Beginners

In 1993, Bill Moyers produced a video shown on Public Television called "Healing and the Mind." In that presentation, an elderly Taiji master said that it took him ten years to experience qi. I considered ten years to be excessively long because, with a few exceptions, I find that my students usually experience qi right away with an exercise taught me by Harvey Sober. Because we have experienced qi since before birth, we tend to disregard it like the fish who says, "Water, what's water?" When two people combine their qi, there is a synergistic effect that can elevate the sensation of qi above the threshold of awareness.

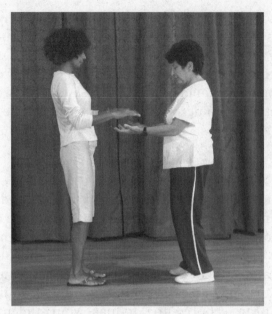

Fig. 13-1. *An exercise to augment the experiencing of qi.*

Sober's exercise involves two people facing each other in a 50-50 stance with knees partly bent (see Fig. 13-1). Both people extend their arms in front of their bodies, one person with palms down and the other with palms up. The palms of each person face the palms of the other. Thus, both people are as if holding two balls, each about four or five inches in diameter.

Testing Students

Periodically having students individually show their movements to the rest of the class and the teacher can be done formally or informally. The formal method has the advantage that it prompts students to practice more and to learn to overcome shyness. But such formality can also discourage a student who learns more slowly. Whether formally or informally, it is very important for the teacher to devote full attention to a student if only for a limited period of time. The rest of the students can watch and learn by formulating their own ideas of what needs work, and they benefit by hearing the teacher's corrections of the student who is "on stage."

Rate of Teaching Movements

My motto is, "It's better to do a small number of movements well than a much larger number of movements less well." The inculcation of the principles is more important than doing a lot of different movements. Therefore, I tend to teach slowly and thoroughly. If a student can learn movements faster by using a videotape or whatever reason, I try to find a way to move that student ahead. But I show most beginners movements at a slow rate and go over them again and again.

Generally, the younger students are, the faster movements can be taught. Teenagers learn very fast but seldom have the patience to go over the same movement numerous times. Elderly people tend to learn much more slowly and require and appreciate frequent repetition.

Student Discouragement After the Second Class

After the second class of a beginner's series, some students become very discouraged and never return. It is often the case that beginning students expect that learning Taiji will be easy and feel that if they are struggling with the beginning movements it means something is wrong. I try to head off such discouragement during the first few classes and especially at the end of those classes by giving "pep talks," emphasizing that Taiji is a very difficult art and that everyone in the class is doing well. Sometimes, I talk of my own difficulties when I was a beginner and say how glad I am that I did not let any discouragement deter me. However, despite all of my encouragement, there are frequently beginners who do not return after the second class.

ADMINISTRATIVE DETAILS

Contacting Students Who Miss Two or More Classes

When I started teaching Taiji, I was presented with a dilemma when a student missed two classes in a row. Usually, a student who misses two successive classes does not return. Should I telephone this student or not? I decided that a student's privacy should be honored, and I refrained from making any calls. At one point, one of my students missed two successive classes, and I felt that she was discouraged and frustrated. I called her and gave her a pep talk—not because I feared losing her as a student but because I truly felt that she was making a mistake in stopping. After my encouragement, she came back to class with renewed enthusiasm. She became quite proficient in all the forms I taught at that time. Eventually she went on to start her own classes with much success and even gave special classes for AIDS patients.

Since this experience, I have called a few of my students but only when I felt that doing so was in the interest of the student or in enhancing the community of learning of the class—not for selfish purposes.

Giving Certificates

I find that giving students certificates for finishing a form (empty-hand, broadsword, double-edged sword, etc.) is a valuable way of acknowledging students' progress and of inspiring beginners. I use a high-quality 32-lb résumé-bond paper and lay it out and word it along the lines of a university diploma.

TEACHING TAIJI PUSH-HANDS

Cooperative Practice. It is crucial to establish an atmosphere of cooperation right from the start. Competitive practice stunts students' growth and can lead to injuries. Doing push-hands competitively, with the primary goal to win, leads to students "forsaking the far for the near." That is, they tend to rely on anything that will work to get the upper hand rather than on cultivating the correct principles. Winning gives immediate satisfaction that quickly evaporates, but inculcating an important principle provides benefits that grow and last forever. In my practice, I try to repeatedly remind myself that every moment is an opportunity to reinforce and learn the principles. Playing to "win by any means" squanders that opportunity.

MAKING CHANGES IN THE TAIJI FORM

A recent development is the use of the word *new*. *New and improved* appears on all manner of consumer items from food to computers. For example, publishing companies purposely "improve" textbooks used in high schools by revising them with distracting pictures, boldface, color type, and things of an entertaining rather than educational nature. The motive behind creating a new edition is to make the previous edition appear obsolete so that last year's books are thrown away rather than used again. Planned obsolescence is built into all manner of goods, which results in our running out of landfill sites.

Some changes, however, are beneficial and even necessary, and few people would suggest that authors write books using typewriters or that people wash laundry on washboards in laundry sinks. Therefore, the question of what change is appropriate arises and is of special importance in teaching Taiji. Here is a quote of Professor Zheng's words on change:[89]

"Under three situations one cannot make changes:
1. If your ability does not reach a certain level, you cannot make changes.
2. If your knowledge is not deep enough, you cannot make changes.
3. If your skill is not polished well, you cannot make changes.

Under three situations one must make change:
1. If you have learned everything from your teacher, you must change.
2. If you have comprehended the ancient philosophy, you must change.
3. If you have run out of the passion in your teaching, you must change.

A greater talent has greater changes; A lesser talent has fewer changes. For those who don't know how to change, it is because their talent and knowledge are not capable. I have never heard of a talented person who did not make changes; I have never seen a person succeed who insisted on changing the unchangeable."

The only way that Taiji can grow and evolve is if students surpass their teachers. The art will deteriorate if students strive to be clones of their teachers. There is no middle ground.

It is important for beginners to do things exactly as taught even though they have an equivalent or seemingly "better" way. As a physics teacher, I know that there are always students who want to do the problem their way. I say, "I can do the problem your way. Can you do it mine? Only when you can do a problem all the different ways are you in a position to judge which way is best." It is best for beginning Taiji students not to "do their own thing." Instead, they should try to do exactly as taught. Of course, asking why it is done that way is totally appropriate, and a good teacher will either know the answer or attempt to find it.

Later, after doing things the teacher's way for a sufficient time, there should be cautious experimentation. After developing a conceptual framework that encompasses an understanding of variations, they can be slowly incorporated.

---

89. From http://www.wuweitaichi.com/articles/Professor_Cheng_Words.htm, *The Tao of Taijiquan*, by Sheng-lun Culture & Publishing Co., Taipei, Taiwan, ISBN 957-9273-02-2, 1985, Translated by David Chen, 1999, p. 221.

Note that there is a difference between making changes in your own practice in private and in teaching these changes to beginners. In an advanced practitioner's private practice, it is valuable to experiment with all manner of variations. It is appropriate to introduce these private changes in class only after they have stood the test of time and have been corroborated by teachers and other practitioners. It is your duty to inform students that you have made changes and what those changes are and why.

MONETARY CONSIDERATIONS

Vocation or Avocation?

True teachers regard teaching primarily as a means of sharing their insights, growth, and joy of experiencing. Such teachers are so excited about learning that they yearn to see others have a corresponding experience. Of course, a good teacher should also receive monetary remuneration as well as the self-development riches of sharing with others. But, in my view, such remuneration should be a by-product rather than a primary goal.

I know several experienced Taiji teachers who decided to quit their professional jobs to teach Taiji as a primary source of income. All of them have been successful and offer their students a lot—but not without paying a price. What I am referring to is the need to commercialize their art in various ways: selling uniforms and tee shirts, charging extra fees for registration and testings, selling nutritional supplements, selling long-term contracts for classes, etc. Sending children to college, paying a mortgage, and supporting a decent lifestyle all create pressure for sustaining a constant flow of income.

My personal preference has been to maintain my original profession to support myself and teach Taiji as a source of growth and supplemental income. That way, when enrollment fluctuates to a temporary low, I do not worry. I feel no need to give a sales pitch to a potential student or hold on to students when it is time for them to move on.

> *Wealth, like happiness, is never attained when sought after directly. It comes as a by-product of providing a useful service.*
>
> —Henry Ford

How Much to Charge?

The amount teachers charge depends on the region, the economy, and personal preferences. Some teachers who are well-heeled charge nothing for their classes. Most teachers charge nothing for the first trial class. The cost of a series of classes will not be the determining factor for most potential students, but it will for some. My preference is to expose Taiji to as many people as possible without feeling taken advantage of monetarily.

Consider that should your deductions be greater than your income for three out of five years, IRS may declare your teaching Taiji a hobby, which means that you will be expected to declare your earnings but never again be able to deduct your expenses.

Charge by the Month or by the Series?

Each method has advantages and disadvantages. Charging by the month has the advantage that all students pay at the same time, which makes it unnecessary to keep track of when each student needs to pay. But how do you charge if a new student comes in during the month? Do you prorate? Also, some months have four weekly meeting times and others have five. Furthermore, if a class is canceled because of snowstorm or other reason, is that class credited to students? If so, how? Finally, if a student goes on vacation or is sick for a prolonged period, I feel it unfair to charge. Charging for an eight- or ten-week series when a student begins requires more time in checking and updating records but is much more flexible.

There are different problems with charging for a series rather than by the month. One problem arises when a student misses the first class of the next series. Whereas it is awkward to start that series with a missed class, I remind myself that I am paying for the space whether or not the student comes and, therefore, do not credit that student with that single missed class. Whatever your policy is, it is good to have a printed sheet documenting your payment polices that you can give to students at the outset (see Payment Policies, below).

What about a "walk-on" fee? If students want to pay by the class, I take the series fee, divide that by one fewer than the number of classes per series, add $1 to that, and round off to the nearest dollar. For example, if the price for a ten-week series is $100, then the walk-on fee would be $(100 \div 9) + 1 = \$12$.

Payment Policies

To avoid misunderstandings, I give each beginning student a copy of the following policies:

1. **General**. Future revisions of the polices described herein will not apply to a student's series currently in progress but will start with the next series. Moreover, these polices do not apply to special classes such as broadsword, double-edged sword, nutrition, etc. The policies for these classes will be announced when they are offered.

2. **Payment**. The fee for each eight-week series of empty-hand form classes is \$XX[90] (or, equivalently, \$YY for a ten-week series), paid in advance. There will be no refunds once a series has started. The spouse (or equivalent), siblings, parents, and children of a student taking an eight- or ten-week series can each attend that series at half price, payable at the start of that series. A student who has finished the form and wants to pay by the class (instead of committing to a series) can do so at \$ZZ[91] per class attended. Special arrangements will be considered for students who find it difficult to pay the cost of classes.

3. **Additional Classes**. A student who has paid for a series can, with Robert Chuckrow's permission, come to additional classes on the same level during that series. There will be a \$6 charge per person for each additional class attended. There is no charge for a make-up class.

4. **Credit for Missed Classes**. If the teacher cancels a class, an additional class is credited to a student who has paid for a series involving that class. No credit will be given for classes of a series that are held but are missed by a student except as follows: A student who misses two or more consecutive classes because of illness is credited with one fewer than the number of classes missed. A vacationing student will similarly be credited but only if Robert Chuckrow is told about the vacation at least one week in advance.

Giving Scholarships to Needy Students

When students indicate an inability to pay for classes, I tell them to pay only an amount they are able to. I tell them to think of it as a scholarship and emphasize that they are not the first to be given that offer. I make that offer without any expectation that I will be reimbursed later, but often I am reimbursed in ways I never expected. One student on scholarship gave me free massages, another helped me rebuild my front staircase, and another made me a beautiful leather attaché case that I use to this day. At the very least, the presence of a devoted student usually enhances the community of learning of the class.

---

90. XX, the eight-week fee, will depend on factors such as what others of your skill level charge in your area. The equivalent ten-week fee, $YY = 1.25\ XX$.
91. $ZZ = (YY \div 9) + 1$.

By the same token, students who are willing to help a teacher by taking over classes in the teacher's absence, or by offering other skills, will often get non-monetary benefits such as an opportunity to teach on their own.

Negotiating a Salary When Teaching for Others

There are a number of factors to take into account when negotiating a salary. One consideration is the lack of charge for the space. Another consideration is the likelihood that some of the students will eventually move into your private classes. If the traveling distance is large, you will spend more time and use more gasoline, and it is less likely that students will eventually travel to classes in your area. Often, a free membership is a fringe benefit of teaching at a fitness club.

A final consideration is whether you will be paid as an employee or a consultant. As an employee, you are very limited in what you can deduct on your income taxes, whereas, as a consultant, you can deduct transportation and many other costs. However, if you make a profit as a consultant, in addition to paying social security taxes for yourself, you will also be required to pay the employer's portion.

PROTECTING YOURSELF

Insurance

Whereas it is very unlikely that a Taiji teacher will be the defendant in a law suit arising from negligent injury to a student, it is still wise to have at least one-million dollars of liability insurance. An umbrella policy is not expensive and may even lower your automobile and homeowner's insurance payments because the umbrella policy will cover some of that liability. Of course, you need to tell the insurance company issuing an umbrella policy that you are teaching Taiji, but if frequent classes are held at your home, the policy may not be offered.

Keeping Records

It is essential to keep accurate track of student information, payments, and attendance. I use a word-processing program to create a file containing the name, address, telephone number(s), starting date, and email address of each student. I then use the "print merge" feature to create 4-inch by 6-inch index cards (rotate the color each year) with the calendar of that year and all of the student's information.

It is very important to keep track of payments received and IRS deductions: cost of advertising, education (classes and workshops you may take plus transportation there and back), car expenses (including advertising transportation), supplies, depreciation of equipment, teaching-related gratuities, Internet-access fee, laundry and cleaning, parking and tolls, telephone, postage (including that for advertising), printing and copying, cost of professional affiliation, subscriptions to related publications, rent on space for classes taught, repair of equipment, tax-preparation fee (including transportation there and back), and work-related meals. It is best to keep computerized records that are updated with each expenditure and payment received

Whenever a student pays me, I tuck that check or cash under the rubber band holding the class cards. When I get home, I immediately enter the information on that student's class card and in my computer. It is embarrassing to forget that a student has already paid me or that a student's tuition is past due.

Similarly, whenever I make a deductible expenditure, I enter that information into my computer at first opportunity. I store all receipts in a file folder in a fireproof box.

Having Students Sign a Waiver and Release

A waiver of an adult student's right to sue, signed by him or her, will not in itself hold up in court. As my lawyer told me, "Either you are negligent or you are not." Nevertheless, having students sign a waiver is of value. By signing such a waiver, (1) students will be more aware of their responsibility to do things safely, (2) be less likely to sue if injured during practice, and (3) find it harder to assert that they were unaware of the dangers of the class should a suit be brought.

Of course, the teacher and those who assist in teaching should at all times be very careful about the well-being of all students. I always tell a new student, "If you feel that what I ask you to do may not be a good idea for you to do, abstain from that movement no matter what I may say." When a student complains of pain, I always advise that student to rest or do things more gently.

Recently, an elderly student of mine suddenly began to act as though he were drunk. He could barely stand and needed to lean on a wall for support. I immediately called 911 while other students brought a chair and prevented the ailing man from falling. EMS came, and one of them routinely asked the man if he were taking a certain class of pharmaceuticals that could have caused the problem. To my relief, the condition *was* caused by those pharmaceuticals—not Qigong or Taiji.

I have assembled the sample waiver shown on the next page from various waivers that I have signed as a student. I have my students sign this waiver if I teach them push-hands. This particular waiver is only an example. You should consult a lawyer before using it.

Sample Flyer

A sample of a flyer that I designed for advertising my classes is shown on the page after the waiver.

Waiver and Release

I, _____, residing at, _____

_____

wish to participate in the training presented by _____.

    I hereby represent that I am physically and emotionally fit to engage in martial arts instructional training and acknowledge that I understand that this training may include vigorous physical movement on my part and on the part of training partners, will involve body contact with training partners, and could expose me to the risk of bodily injury. I further acknowledge that by entering into the training activity provided, I could be exposed to a risk of personal injury arising out of possible negligence or unavoidable accident due to the very nature of the self-defense arts being taught. Moreover, I hereby acknowledge that I am fully responsible to use or apply or not to use or apply, at my discretion, all or any portion of the ideas and/or information I may receive while studying with _____.

    I hereby acknowledge that _____ has made it clear, and I fully realize that, during the training, I will always and at all times have the option of withdrawing from participation in any exercise or technique and that it is my personal responsibility to decide which exercises and techniques I will participate in.

    By signing this agreement, it is my stated intention to knowingly assume all risks involved in participation in this training and, for myself and my heirs, executors, administrators, successors, assigns, and personal representatives, release and discharge _____, his family, successors, or assigns from any and all claims, costs, liabilities, expenses, or judgments, including attorney's fees and court costs ("Claims") arising out of my participation in T'AI CHI CH'UAN classes or from any illness, injury, or loss resulting therefrom, and I hereby agree to indemnify and hold
harmless from and against any and all such Claims except Claims proximately caused by his gross negligence or willful misconduct. This agreement cannot be modified orally. A waiver of any provision of this agreement shall not be construed as a modification of any other provision or as a consent to any other provision or as a consent to any other subsequent waiver or modification.

    I hereby execute and deliver this Agreement as of the date written below my signature.

_____
Signature of Student

_____
Date

Tai Chi

with Robert Chuckrow, Ph.D.

Saturdays, 9:30 A.M. at Trinity Church,
7 S. Highland Ave. (Rte. 9 & Ellis Pl.), Ossining, NY.

About Tai Chi:

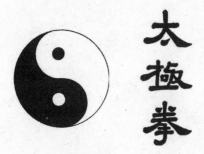

About the Teacher:

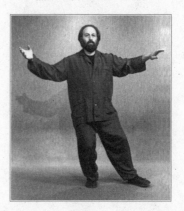

Tai Chi is a meditative exercise based on Taoist philosophy and other centuries-old Chinese principles of health, spirituality, and self-defense. Its natural, relaxed movements promote inner calm and improve self-awareness, balance, and coordination. Recently published studies have confirmed that those who do Tai Chi have improved blood pressure and are much less susceptible to falls and their resulting injuries.

Because of its richness, Tai Chi is called "the pearl of Chinese knowledge and culture."

Dr. Chuckrow has taught Tai Chi extensively and has authored five books. One of his three books on Tai Chi was a finalist in the Independent Publisher Book Awards in the health/medicine category. He has studied Tai Chi, Ch'i Kung, and other movement and healing arts since 1970.

Chuckrow holds a Ph.D. in experimental physics from NYU and has taught physics at NYU, The Cooper Union, and other schools for the past forty-three years.

Beginners can start at any time, and the first trial class is free.

Information: www.bestweb.net/~taichi

14

Miscellaneous

ROMANIZATION OF CHINESE WORDS

There have been seven different ways of Romanizing Chinese words during the time period between 1912 and 1958.[92] At present, the pinyin (*spell sound*) system is prevalent and lends itself well to converting Chinese words spelled in Latin characters to Chinese characters to be set in type on a computer. Missing in most books that have Chinese words in pinyin (including this book) are the five tones, which distinguish one pinyin word from a host of others. Pronouncing a Chinese word correctly without including the appropriate tone will usually result in a Chinese speaker completely misunderstanding what you are saying.

The Chinese character for each word, however, is distinct. When converting a word spelled in pinyin to its specific Chinese character when using a computer with the appropriate software, the pinyin word is typed in, and a number of characters all having that pinyin spelling appear on the screen. The appropriate character can then be selected and incorporated as text. More recently, a system of achieving Chinese characters digitally involves drawing each character on a touch pad with a stylus. The character then appears on the computer screen.

One of the difficulties with pinyin is that its spelling of words tends to be more arbitrary than phonetic. For example the word *qi* might be thought to be pronounced *kwee*, but it is actually pronounced *chee*. It is therefore necessary to learn how to pronounce each of the sixty consonants and vowels that are utilized as basic sounds. Once you learn to pronounce

---

92. See http://www.white-clouds.com/iclc/cliej/cl4ao.htm for a historical perspective of Romanization of Chinese words.

these basic sounds, along with the five tones, you can look up an English word in a Chinese-English, English-Chinese dictionary[93] and be able to pronounce it in Chinese.

The older Wade-Giles[94] system of Romanization is more phonetic than pinyin but does not lend itself to setting Chinese into type on a computer. The Wade-Giles system is less precise in bringing out subtle differences in pronunciation. One of the most obvious features of Wade-Giles is the use of apostrophes after a consonant to denote that the consonant is not sounded, e.g., *ch'i* (pronounced *chee*) compared to *chi* (pronounced *jee*).

A document written in Chinese characters is extremely compact. In the United Nations, where all speeches are printed in each language, the Chinese version takes much less paper than the English version does.

DOES DOING TAIJI EXERCISE EVERY MUSCLE IN YOUR BODY?

When I started doing Taiji, a friend asked me the above question. My skill level at the time caused me to think that the question was silly because, in Taiji, we are not interested in muscular strength. Now I know that to move with unified strength not only means using every muscle, but it also means using every muscle in a highly beneficial manner that stimulates circulation of oxygenated blood and qi.

When you practice unified strength in Qigong and in the Taiji form, over a period of time, you will get much benefit from naturally increasing the level of muscular action one "grain at a time." Practicing Qigong or Taiji this way will eventually make you very strong but not in the conventional way.

IS SWEATING DURING FORM AND PUSH-HANDS PRACTICE UNDESIRABLE?

If a student began to sweat while doing the form or push-hands, Professor Zheng would make that student stop and sit down, saying, "Rest." Sweating—even in hot weather—was considered a sign that you were doing something wrong. On the other hand, some teachers take sweating

---

93. Especially useful is the *Concise English-Chinese Chinese-English Dictionary*, Oxford University Press, 1999.
94. See http://www.ibiblio.org/chinesehistory/contents/c06s01.html for cross-referencing many Chinese words from Wade-Giles to Pinyin and from Pinyin to Wade-Giles.

while doing the form to be a *good* sign. Since, in the early 1970s, Zheng was emphasizing total relaxation rather than strength-building, his approach is certainly understandable. However, for someone working on building correct strength, sweating may be a good sign.

A few times, I have perspired profusely when the qi from doing the form was extremely strong. Perhaps sweating can result from more than one reason. Certainly, contractive muscular action takes more energy, which is undesirable. But extension opens up everything in the body, which *is* desirable. Thus, I keep an open mind on this subject and do not know the answer.

ASKING QUESTIONS

It is essential to be careful whom you ask a question because the answer has power. The more credentials a person has, the more power the answer tends to have. If the answer is one that leads you astray, you will have difficulty in shedding its influence. The solution is not to stop asking questions of those who you think can be helpful; it just requires maintaining an optimal balance between inquisitiveness, an open mind, self-reliance, and healthy skepticism.

TO ANALYZE OR NOT?

There is a tendency among some Taiji students not to analyze their movements scientifically, in terms of physics, skeletal and muscular anatomy, physiology, and psychology. These students are content to repeat their movements until the correct way of doing things develops. They feel that analyzing things may give momentary dividends but limit things in the long run. As one who owes most of his progress to applying scientific analysis to movement, I am, of course, a proponent of doing so. Why not bring all appropriate tools into the situation?

> *Every tool you try to get along without, you pay for in the long run.*
> —Henry Ford

VISUALIZATION OF SKELETAL RELATIONSHIPS

In 1973, I took a course in Ideokinesis with André Bernard (1924–2003). The purpose of the course was to understand skeletal relationships and to be able to visualize your own bones as you move. Students were required to trace drawings of bones from an art-anatomy book. Bernard then gave us movement exercises to do while visualizing the changing relationships of a group of bones in our bodies. Since taking that course, I have been able to visualize my skeleton as if seeing a continuous X-ray of myself as I move.

I am convinced that understanding and visualizing skeletal relationships is important for correcting errors in skeletal alignment. Following Bernard's example, I periodically bring a small, 18-inch-tall, flexible, realistic, plastic skeleton (see Fig. 14-1) to Taiji classes and use it to point out various details to my students. I also encourage my students to obtain an anatomy book and study the drawings.

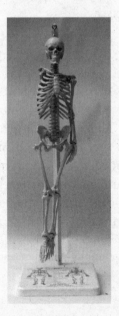

Fig. 14-1. *An 18-inch-tall plastic skeleton. One arm was lost after it was removed for demonstration purposes. This skeleton is available from Premier Medical Products (http://premieremedical.safeshopper.com/14/240.htm?209).*

COMPARISON OF ZHENG'S SHORT FORM
WITH OTHER YANG-STYLE FORMS

Order of Movements

There is only one departure in the order of the movements of Zheng's short form from that of the long form. In the short form "Downward Single Whip" and "Golden Cock Left and Right" occur before "Fair Lady Works Shuttles" instead of afterward, in the long form.

Differences in Interpretation

One seemingly exclusive characteristic of Zheng's short form occurs when the right foot takes a "side step" in front of the left foot in the transition from the second to third corner in "Four Corners." Many practitioners disparage such stepping, saying that it is not in accordance with Taiji principles. Such stepping also occurs in other arts such as Bagua and Ninjutsu (the Ninja call side stepping *yoko aruki*). A side step *is* in accord with the Taiji principles if done naturally, utilizing the natural swing of the leg resulting from the large sideways shifting of the body in that transition.

Differences in 100% Stances and in Transitions in 70-30 Stances

It appears that Zheng changed the angle of the weighted foot in 100% stances from 45° to the forward foot to 90° to the forward foot. Examples are "White Crane Spreads Wings," "Raise Hands," and "Kick with Heel." This change was apparently made to encourage us to open our thigh joints more. Others who studied with Zheng's teacher, Yang Cheng-fu, preset the rear foot to 45° with the forward foot prior to attaining certain 70-30 and 100% stances.

Consider, for example, both ways of making the transition from "Ward off Left" to "Ward off Right." In Zheng's style, weight is shifted 100% onto the left foot, which remains pointed in the starting direction, arbitrarily defined as north. The right foot then steps east, a shoulder width from the left foot. After the weight shifts 70% onto the right foot, the body turns to face east, pivoting the left foot 45° on its heel. By contrast, other disciples of Yang Cheng-fu make this transition as follows: From "Ward off Left," weight is shifted 100% onto the right foot, and the body turns to the right, pivoting the left foot 45° on its heel. The weight is then shifted back

100% onto the left foot, and the right foot then steps east, a shoulder width from the left foot. The weight shifts 70% onto the right foot, but the body does not turn because it already faces east.

A similar difference occurs in making transitions from 70-30 stances to 100% stances.

FOOTWEAR

For most Taiji practitioners, Kung Fu slippers, which can be easily bought,[95] are entirely adequate. However, practitioners whose feet are very wide or very narrow cannot so easily be fitted. It is possible to obtain custom-made Kung Fu slippers by sending an outline of your foot to certain manufacturers in Taiwan. However, it is not hard to make your own slippers that are just as good (see Fig. 14-2).

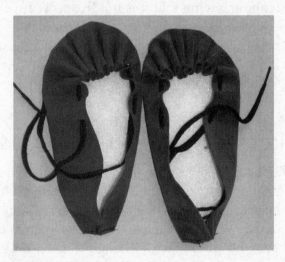

Fig. 14-2. *A photograph of slippers made by the author for his two-year-old grandson.*

To proceed, make an outline of your foot with full weight on it. Cut out the outline and measure the length. Divide that length by the length of the outline in Fig. 14-3. Multiply that quotient by 100%, and use a computer graphics program or photocopier to enlarge the pattern by that factor. If using a photocopier, you may need to make a succession of enlargements to achieve the final size. For example, if the length of your foot is 13

---

95. Available from Asian World of Martial Arts, 9400 Ashton Road, Philadelphia, PA 19114, www.awma.com.

inches and the length of the foot in Fig. 14-3 is 3 inches, the enlargement factor would be 13 ÷ 3 = 4.33. Multiplying 4.33 by 100% yields 433%. Make a 200% copy of Fig. 14-3 and then another 200% copy of the first copy. That will have enlarged the pattern in Fig. 12-3 by a factor of four. Next make a copy of the second (400%) copy with an enlargement of 433% ÷ 4 = 108%. Now check the size of the foot outline of this copy with that of your foot. Once you achieve the correct length, using a pencil, reduce or enlarge the outer outline proportionally.

When you have a pattern of approximately the right size (the size is not really critical), cut out the outer shape, and use this pattern for tracing the outline on real or artificial leather.

Choose leather that is supple enough to have 180° folds in it. You can check the strength of leather by making a one-inch-long slit in a place where the leather will not be used. Insert both forefingers into the slit and pull the leather apart. The leather should be strong enough to withstand quite a bit of force without tearing.

Once the leather is cut to shape and size, punch the holes, and sew edges marked "B" in Fig. 14-3 together, edges marked "C" together, and then edges marked "A" together. Note that the smooth side of the leather is on the outside. You can obtain a pair of fleece insoles, cut them to the outline of your foot, and place them inside. If necessary, insoles can be glued using a dab of rubber cement.

PRACTICE: THE RIGHT TIME AND THE RIGHT PLACE

Practicing regularly raises the probability that you will be in the correct modality when an important insight is ready to percolate into your awareness.

> *The hours of folly are measur'd by the clock, but of wisdom: no clock can measure.*
> —William Blake, *The Marriage of Heaven and Hell*, "Proverbs of Hell."

This quote can be used as a reply to someone who asks, "How long have you studied Taiji?"

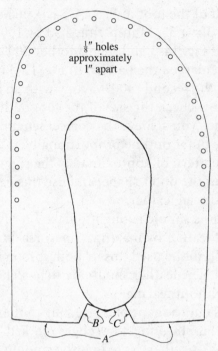

Fig. 14-3. *The pattern for the type of slippers shown in the previous figure. An approximate pattern can be made for your foot by photocopying the above pattern to a scale that enlarges the center foot-tracing to roughly match the tracing of your foot.*

TEACHERS: THE RIGHT TIME AND THE RIGHT PLACE

It is not uncommon for people who have collected possessions for a lifetime to suddenly give their treasures away. So it is with some teachers who have taught sparingly, waiting for the right person to come along. At a certain point, when they see that they might die with their knowledge, they become more willing to share it. It is always good when you are the person who is present at that time.

"MUSCLE MEMORY"

Reference is often made to the benefit of repetitive practice on "muscle memory." The implication of such a characterization is that muscles have an intelligence of their own. Without the receiving, sending, and processing of neural sense data by the brain, muscles may exhibit genetically preprogrammed reflexes but are essentially incapable of fine-motor responses.

One of the main precepts of Taiji is to eliminate habitual, reflex responses to situations and replace such responses with moment-by-moment ones that are finely tuned to each individual situation. Whereas it is true that appropriate, timely responses occur seemingly without conscious thought and, sometimes, even without awareness, such responses, nevertheless, occur by means of refined neural processes.

An offhand way of speaking is sometimes of value, but when dealing with a complex and elusive art such as Taiji, it is essential not to characterize processes in a manner that can be misleading. Therefore, we should refrain from using the term *muscle memory*.

Persistence

In 1970, I bought a full-concert, double-manual harpsichord kit (Fig. 14-4). I fully intended to build it in record time. I spent part of that summer working on it. Then things came along that caused me to put it aside. The unfinished harpsichord lay on its spine in my living room for the next four years. When I moved from an apartment to a house, the harpsichord found a new location to lie on its side, which it did for another eight years. Each time I saw the unfinished instrument, I decided that building it had to wait until I had the time.

In the summer of 1982, I thought, if I do not do anything, I will never build that harpsichord, but if I do a little bit every day, it will eventually get built. By the end of that summer, the harpsichord was completely built (Fig. 14-5).

Recently, I saw the following inscription and its translation mounted on the wall of a New York City subway corridor: *Gutta cavat lapidem, non vi, sed saepe cadendo* (dripping water hollows out a stone, not with force but by falling often).

The Importance of Small Things

Recently, I heard a radio interview with a concentration-camp survivor of the Nazi holocaust. He said that the guards would taunt starving prisoners by throwing eggshells at them. He collected the eggshells, salvaged the membranes, and fed them to the children. He felt that that small amount of nutrition made the difference between some of them starving to death

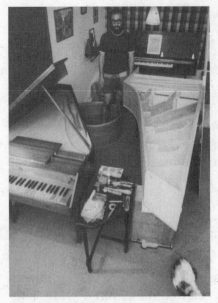

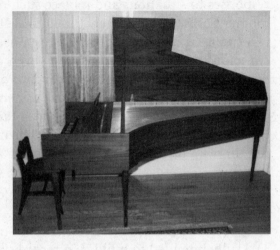

Fig. 14-4. *The author in 1970, standing (with one foot inside a roll of veneer) next to a harpsichord and clavichord, each of which he built from Zuckermann kits, and an unfinished double-manual harpsichord from a Hubbard kit that he was in the process of building. His cat, Chambis, (in foreground) naps peacefully.*

Fig. 14-5. *A view of the double-manual harpsichord that the author completed in 1982.*

and not. Herbert Shelton said that the minute amount of energy expended in chewing a stick of gum might mean the difference between life and death for a patient who is barely holding on to life.

Similarly, in a self-defense situation, a very small injury, error in judgment, or wrong movement can mean the difference between life and death. In most cases, it never comes to that, so we do not recognize the consequences of our actions. However, the more finely tuned and aware we become (through meditation, introspection, and critical thinking), the more we are able to see the far-reaching effects of the seemingly small things that occur in our daily lives.

TECHNIQUES VERSUS ILLUSTRATIONS

One of the hallmarks of Taijiquan is that there are no techniques as in other martial arts such as, for example, Karate. It is said that the basis for study in Karate is the development of strength, speed, and technique. In Karate the kata (forms) are composed of fighting moves, each of which is a technique intended for countering a specific attack or mounting an attack. The scientific nature of Karate makes it much more easily systematized, and a given skill level in self-defense is much more quickly achieved in Karate than in Taijiquan.

In Taijiquan the movements of the form are more for *illustrating* an application in a self-defense situation. That is, warriors of centuries ago came back from a battle and told their colleagues how they successfully defended certain attacks. Then, those sequences were practiced as exercises, not with the expectation that those same situations would necessarily occur again but to inculcate principles of correct movement. Of course, those who were unsuccessful in defending against an attack explained *those* details to others—if they survived.

In repetitive practice of Taijiquan applications with a partner, it is necessary for both partners to stick to their roles. But if one person deviates and his or her partner responds the same way as before, that response is now inappropriate.

ONE SIZE FITS ALL

We are told how many glasses of water to drink per day, how many servings to eat of each of the food groups, how long to take a nap, and other arbitrary amounts of things that should be done the same way by everyone. Actually, someone who works at a desk in an air-conditioned office has different water needs than a person who does physical labor all day in the hot sun. In fact, each person's needs vary from day to day and even from moment to moment.

There is little mention of becoming attuned to one's own body and the effects of things and their amounts. Often, the scientific principles involved are not mentioned, and even when they are, the science is usually manipulated for the purpose of selling a particular product such as bran, red wine, green tea, or chocolate.

One of the goals of practicing Taiji is to learn the effects of everything—every thought, utterance, action, movement, and substance ingested, whether it be food that is nutritious or laced with artificial flavor, artificial color, preservatives, etc. Of course, it is impossible to know everything on our own, and that is where science and the experience of others are important ingredients in helping to sort out the effects of things.

Thus, Taiji players should be the least likely to have a one-size-fits-all mentality.

Content Versus Outer Appearance

We live in a world where, in many realms, appearance takes precedence over content. Because of industrialization, many things have become very complicated. At the same time, few people have the critical faculties to understand details or probe beneath the surface. Therefore, most people judge things superficially, by their immediate visual affect.

There are many differences in ways of doing everything including Taiji. Think of how many ways there are to prepare eggs: soft-boiled, poached, hard-boiled, Benedictine, Florentine, sunny-side-up, once-over-lightly, coddled, scrambled, deviled, quiche, and all the different types of omelets. China is a very large country, with many different types of weather, terrain, clothing, occupations, transportation, and general conditions. Taiji is based on thousands of years of Chinese martial arts, philosophy, and knowledge of healing. Therefore, it is totally out of keeping with the principles and essence of Taiji to disparage another's way of doing Taiji movement just because it looks different. Instead, it is better to find out why the person does it differently before criticizing. If the different way embodies the Taiji principles, then learn from that difference. Only if the different way is haphazard or in violation of the principles, should it be rejected.

Studying With a Teacher Whose Interpretation is Different From That of a Prior Teacher

Early on in my Taiji studies, I was studying concurrently with Zheng Manqing and William C.C. Chen. Chen had been a student of Zheng when in China and started his own school when he came to the United States. There were minor differences between these two masters' forms. One difference was that Chen put back some of the movements of the long form. Other differences were how the movements were interpreted.

On one occasion, when I asked Chen about an interpretive difference, he said, "That is the way Zheng originally taught it to me in China. He has since changed it." On another occasion, Chen said, "I did it the way Zheng taught me for twenty years and then changed it to a way that I consider to be more correct." When I asked him which way I should do it, he said, "Practice both ways, and you'll find out." I took Chen's comment to heart and started to let the movements tell me how they should be done rather than copying one or another teacher.

STORY OF THE MUSIC PALACE THEATER

When I first started studying Taiji in the early 1970s, I frequented several nearby theaters that almost exclusively featured martial-arts movies. These were the Music Palace Theater, the Pagoda Theater and the Sun Sing Theater. The Music Palace, next door to the *Shr Jung* Taiji school at 87 Bowery, closed in 2000 and was torn down afterward. There was another theater in Chinatown, the Gouverneur, which I never had occasion to patronize.

One weekday afternoon, I was watching a martial-arts movie in the Music Palace. Suddenly, I was gripped with intense fear that had nothing to do with the events of the movie or anything else I could discern. I immediately left the theater. Once in the sunlight, the fear disappeared completely. I had never experienced an event such as that before and had no idea what caused it.

A few months later, I went to the Music Palace again. Part way through the movie, I was again gripped with fear. I left, knowing then that it was something about the theater and not something wrong with me.

One day, I overheard one of my Taiji classmates talking in a very concerned manner about an "anxiety attack" she had experienced. I asked her, "where were you when it happened?" The reply was, "the Music Palace Theater." I told her of my two experiences and reassured her that there was nothing wrong with her—it was the theater.

Recently, I told my Taiji students the above story. Afterward, one student, who is Chinese, remarked, "I had "goose bumps along my spine while you spoke." He explained that there had long been a rumor in Chinatown that that theater was haunted.

CATEGORIZATION OF MOVEMENTS

Harvey Sober taught me an aid to learning movements, which involves categorizing movements into types. His method is analogous to that used by musicians who are able to reproduce music by hearing it in terms of chord progressions.

Sober compares the movements of any form to a Chinese-restaurant menu: There may be well over a hundred different dishes, but a good many dishes are composed of only several basic ingredients. There is beef with bean sprouts, beef with Chinese vegetables, beef with mushrooms, beef with snow peas, beef with black bean sauce, and beef with broccoli. Then there is chicken with bean sprouts, chicken with Chinese vegetables, chicken with mushrooms, chicken with snow peas, chicken with black bean sauce, and chicken with broccoli. And so on with pork, shrimp, and duofu (tofu). Similarly, the externals of a good many Taiji movements are likewise variations of only several basic ingredients and can be categorized in at least the following ways:

1. In terms of the plane or planes (sagittal, frontal, or horizontal) in which the movement occurs (see Chapter 3 for definitions of these planes).
2. In terms of clockwise or counterclockwise.
3. In terms of parallel or opposite motion of the hands.
4. In terms of two basic movements, namely, "Ward Off" and "Brush Knee." The "Ward Off" movements involve one or both hands *rising* along the front of the body and moving outward whereas the "Brush Knee" movements involve one or both hands *descending* along the front of the body and moving outward. The following is such a categorization of some of the movements in the Taiji form:

Ward Off
- Single Whip
- White Crane
- Cloud Hands
- Four Corners
- Diagonal Flying
- Separate Foot (L & R)
- Parting the Wild Horse's Mane*
- Fan Through the Back*

Brush Knee
- Roll Back
- Strike with Shoulder
- Carry Tiger to Mountain
- Step Back, Ride Tiger
- Strike Tiger on Right (Left)*
- Downward Single Whip
- Repulse Monkey
- Strike Ears With Fists*
- Fan Through the Back*

*These movements are in the long form.

Bibliography

Bragg, Paul C, *The Miracle of Fasting*, Health Science, Box 15000, Santa Anna, CA 92705, 1975.

Carrington, Hereward, *Fasting for Health and Long Life*, Health Research, Mokelumne Hill, CA, 1953.

Chen, William C. C., *Body Mechanics of T'ai Chi Ch'uan*, William C. C. Chen Publisher, New York, NY, 1973.

Chen, William C. C., "William C. C. Chen on Tai Chi Breathing," *T'ai Chi Magazine*, December, 2006.

Cheng Man-ch'ing, *Cheng Tzu's Thirteen Treatises on T'ai Chi Ch'uan*, North Atlantic Books, Berkeley, CA, 1985.

Cheng Man-ch'ing, *T'ai Chi Ch'uan: A Simplified Method of Calisthenics for Health & Self Defense*, North Atlantic Books, Berkeley, CA, 1981 (new edition of the original book, printed in China in 1962).

Chin Fan-siong, *I Liq Chuan*, Chin Family I Liq Chuan Association, P. O. Box 374, Mount Kisco, NY 10549, 2006, ISBN 978-0-9776587-0-1.

Chuckrow, Robert, *Tai Chi Walking*, YMAA Publication Center, Boston, MA, 2002.

Chuckrow, Robert, *The Intelligent Dieter's Guide*, Rising Mist Publications, Briarcliff Manor, NY, 1997.

Chuckrow, Robert, *The Tai Chi Book*, YMAA Publication Center, Boston, MA, 1998.

Concise English-Chinese Chinese-English Dictionary, Oxford University Press, 1999.

De Vries, Arnold, *Therapeutic Fasting*, Chandler Book Co., Los Angeles, CA, 1963. This book is out of print but can be obtained from http://www.soilandhealth.org/copyform.aspx?bookcode=020141.

Duff, Karl J., *Martial Arts & the Law*, Ohara Publications, Burbank. CA, 1985.

Edward R. Shaw, *Physics by Experiment*, Maynard, Merrill, & Co., New York, 1897.

The Essence of T'ai Chi Ch'uan, The Literary Tradition, Edited by Benjamin Pang-jeng Lo et al., North Atlantic Books, Berkeley, CA, 1985.

Galante, Lawrence, *Tai Chi The Supreme Ultimate*, Samuel Weiser, Inc., York Beach, MA, 1981.

Hatsumi, Masaaki and Chambers, Quinton, *Stick Fighting*, Kdansha International Ltd., New York, 1981, ISBN 0-97011-475-1.

Home Firearm Safety, Published By the National Rifle Association of America, 1990.

Jancich, Michael D., *Fighting Folders*, VHS, Paladin Press, PO Box 1307, Boulder, CO 80306, ISBN1-58160-093-3.

Lao Tzu: "My words are easy to understand," Lectures on the Tao Teh Ching by Man-jan Zheng, Translated by Tam C. Gibbs, North Atlantic Books, 1981.

Lee Ying Arng, *Lee's Modifid Tai Chi for Health*, Unicorn Press, P.O. Box 2448, Hong Kong, Distributed by Mclisa Enterprises, P.O. Box 1755, Honolulu, Hawaii 96806, 1968.

Lipman, Ira A., *How to Protect Yourself from Crime*, Contemporary Books, Chicago, IL, 1989.

Montagu, Ashley, *On Being Human*, Hawthorn Books, Inc., New York, 1966.

Ramacharaka, Yogi, *Science of Breath*, Yogi Publication Society, Chicago, IL. 1904, (ISBN 0-911662-00-6), available from Wheman Bros. Hackensack, NJ.

Shaw, Edward R., *Physics by Experiment*, Maynard, Merrill, & Co., New York, 1897.

Shelton, Herbert M., *Fasting and Sunbathing*, Dr. Shelton's Health School, San Antonio, TX, 1963

Shelton, Herbert M., *Fasting Can Save Your Life*, Natural Hygiene Press, Inc., Chicago, IL, 1964.

Smith, Robert W., *Martial Musings: A Portrayal of Martial Arts in the 20th Century*, Via Media Publishing Company, Erie, PA, 1999.

Yang, Jwing-Ming, *Tai Chi Secrets of the Ancient Masters*, YMAA Publication Center, Boston, MA, 1999.

INTERNET SOURCES

http://library.ust.hk/guides/opac/conversion-tables.html.

http://www.bestweb.net/~taichi (author's website)

http://www.ccat.sas.upenn.edu/~nsivin/mm.html, Index to Shiu-Ying Hu, An Enumeration of Chinese Materia Medica, Hong Kong, 1980 (list of TCM pharmacopoeia).

http://www.ccat.sas.upenn.edu/~nsivin/mm.html, Index to Shiu-Ying Hu, An Enumeration of Chinese Materia Medica, Hong Kong, 1980.

http://www.chenzhonghua.com/Articles/Chen%20On%20Peng.htm.

http://www.emedicine.com/ped/byname/apnea-of-prematurity.htm (discussion of fetal breathing).

http://www.geocities.com/meiyingsheng/story.html (story of how Yang Cheng-fu avoided a deadly confrontation and made a friend).

http://www.ibiblio.org/chinesehistory/contents/c06s01.html (discussion of the various "Romanizations" of Chinese words and cross-referencing of them).

http://www.library.ust.hk/guides/opac/conversion-tables.html (list of Pinyin/Wade-Giles conversions).

http://www.sparknotes.com/testprep/books/sat2/math2c/chapter3section3.rhtml (discussion of math S.A.T. preparation).

http://www.taiji-qigong.de/info/articles/jumin_transljin_en.php (discussion of *pengjin*).

http://www.white-clouds.com/iclc/cliej/cl4ao.htm (historical perspective of Romanization of Chinese words).

http://www.wuweitaichi.com/articles/Professor_Cheng_Words.htm, The Tao of Taijiquan, by Sheng-lun Culture & Publishing Co., Taipei, Taiwan, ISBN 957-9273-02-2, 1985, Translated by David Chen, 1999.

Index

Also by Robert Chuckrow . . .

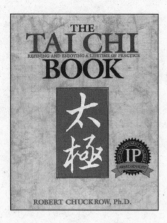

THE TAI CHI BOOK—
Refining and Enjoying a Lifetime of Practice

Robert Chuckrow, Ph.D.
A detailed guide for students who have learned a Tai Chi form and want to know more. It also introduces beginners to the principles behind great Tai Chi, showing you how to use Tai Chi to gain strength in your bones, muscles, and vital organs; how to improve your balance and flexibility; and to achieve remarkable vitality. Includes practice exercises and great ideas for teachers.

208 pages • 126 illus. • ISBN: 1-886969-64-7

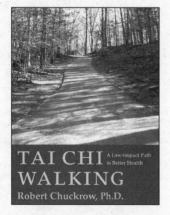

TAI CHI WALKING—A Low-Impact Approach to Better Health
Robert Chuckrow, Ph.D.
For Tai Chi practitioners, walking provides an excellent opportunity to augment, refine, and reinforce Tai Chi principles and bridge the gap between formal practice and everyday life. For non-practitioners, Tai Chi Walking trains us in concepts for improving health, balance, peace of mind, and safety. Highly informative.

160 pages • 40 illus. • ISBN: 1-886969-23-X

BOOKS FROM YMAA

more products available from...

YMAA Publication Center, Inc. 楊氏東方文化出版中心

1-800-669-8892 • ymaa@aol.com • www.ymaa.com

YMAA
PUBLICATION CENTER

VIDEOS FROM YMAA

ADVANCED PRACTICAL CHIN NA — 1	T0061
ADVANCED PRACTICAL CHIN NA — 2	T007X
COMP. APPLICATIONS OF SHAOLIN CHIN NA 1	T386
COMP. APPLICATIONS OF SHAOLIN CHIN NA 2	T394
EIGHT SIMPLE QIGONG EXERCISES FOR HEALTH 2ND ED.	T54X
NORTHERN SHAOLIN SWORD — SAN CAI JIAN & ITS APPLICATIONS	T051
NORTHERN SHAOLIN SWORD — KUN WU JIAN & ITS APPLICATIONS	T06X
NORTHERN SHAOLIN SWORD — QI MEN JIAN & ITS APPLICATIONS	T078
QIGONG: 15 MINUTES TO HEALTH	T140
SHAOLIN LONG FIST KUNG FU — YI LU MEI FU & ER LU MAI FU	T256
SHAOLIN LONG FIST KUNG FU — SHI ZI TANG	T264
SHAOLIN LONG FIST KUNG FU — XIAO HU YAN	T604
SHAOLIN WHITE CRANE GONG FU — BASIC TRAINING 3	T0185
SIMPLIFIED TAI CHI CHUAN — 24 & 48	T329
SUN STYLE TAIJIQUAN	T469
TAI CHI CHUAN & APPLICATIONS — 24 & 4	T485
TAIJI CHIN NA IN DEPTH — 1	T0282
TAIJI CHIN NA IN DEPTH — 2	T0290
TAIJI CHIN NA IN DEPTH — 3	T0304
TAIJI CHIN NA IN DEPTH — 4	T0312
TAIJI WRESTLING — 1	T0371
TAIJI WRESTLING — 2	T038X
TAIJI YIN & YANG SYMBOL STICKING HANDS–YANG TAIJI TRAINING	T580
TAIJI YIN & YANG SYMBOL STICKING HANDS–YIN TAIJI TRAINING	T0177
WILD GOOSE QIGONG	T949
WU STYLE TAIJIQUAN	T477
XINGYIQUAN — 12 ANIMAL FORM	T310

DVDS FROM YMAA

ANALYSIS OF SHAOLIN CHIN NA	D0231
BAGUAZHANG 1,2, & 3 —EMEI BAGUAZHANG	D0649
CHEN STYLE TAIJIQUAN	D0819
CHIN NA IN DEPTH COURSES 1 — 4	D602
CHIN NA IN DEPTH COURSES 5 — 8	D610
CHIN NA IN DEPTH COURSES 9 — 12	D629
EIGHT SIMPLE QIGONG EXERCISES FOR HEALTH	D0037
FIVE ANIMAL SPORTS	D1106
THE ESSENCE OF TAIJI QIGONG	D0215
QIGONG MASSAGE—FUNDAMENTAL TECHNIQUES FOR HEALTH AND RELAXATION	D0592
SHAOLIN KUNG FU FUNDAMENTAL TRAINING 1&2	D0436
SHAOLIN LONG FIST KUNG FU — BASIC SEQUENCES	D661
SHAOLIN SABER — BASIC SEQUENCES	D0616
SHAOLIN STAFF — BASIC SEQUENCES	D0920
SHAOLIN WHITE CRANE GONG FU BASIC TRAINING 1&2	D599
SIMPLE QIGONG EXERCISES FOR ARTHRITIS RELIEF	D0890
SIMPLE QIGONG EXERCISES FOR BACK PAIN RELIEF	D0883
SIMPLIFIED TAI CHI CHUAN	D0630
SUNRISE TAI CHI	D0274
SUNSET TAI CHI	D0760
TAI CHI CONNECTIONS	D0444
TAI CHI ENERGY PATTERNS	D0525
TAI CHI FIGHTING SET—TWO PERSON MATCHING SET	D0509
TAIJI BALL QIGONG COURSES 1&2—16 CIRCLING AND 16 ROTATING PATTERNS	D0517
TAIJI BALL QIGONG COURSES 3&4—16 PATTERNS OF WRAP-COILING & APPLICATIONS	D0777
TAIJI MARTIAL APPLICATIONS — 37 POSTURES	D1057
TAIJI PUSHING HANDS 1&2—YANG STYLE SINGLE AND DOUBLE PUSHING HANDS	D0495
TAIJI PUSHING HANDS 3&4—MOVING SINGLE AND DOUBLE PUSHING HANDS	D0681
TAIJI SABER — THE COMPLETE FORM, QIGONG & APPLICATIONS	D1026
TAIJI & SHAOLIN STAFF - FUNDAMENTAL TRAINING	D0906
TAIJI YIN YANG STICKING HANDS	D1040
TAIJIQUAN CLASSICAL YANG STYLE	D645
TAIJI SWORD, CLASSICAL YANG STYLE	D0452
UNDERSTANDING QIGONG 1 — WHAT IS QI? • HUMAN QI CIRCULATORY SYSTEM	D069X
UNDERSTANDING QIGONG 2 — KEY POINTS • QIGONG BREATHING	D0418
UNDERSTANDING QIGONG 3 — EMBRYONIC BREATHING	D0555
UNDERSTANDING QIGONG 4 — FOUR SEASONS QIGONG	D0562
UNDERSTANDING QIGONG 5 — SMALL CIRCULATION	D0753
UNDERSTANDING QIGONG 6 — MARTIAL QIGONG BREATHING	D0913
WHITE CRANE HARD & SOFT QIGONG	D637

more products available from...

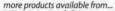

YMAA Publication Center, Inc. 楊氏東方文化出版中心

1-800-669-8892 • ymaa@aol.com • www.ymaa.com

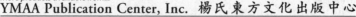